Central Venous Catheters

Central Venous Catheters

Edited by

Helen Hamilton
CBE FRCN RGN

Oxford Radcliffe Hospitals Trust
Oxford, UK

Andrew R. Bodenham
FRCA

Consultant in Anaesthesia and Intensive Care Medicine
Leeds General Infirmary
Leeds, UK

⊛WILEY-BLACKWELL

A John Wiley & Sons, Ltd., Publication

Wiley-Blackwell is an imprint of John Wiley and Sons, formed by the merger of Wiley's global
Scientific, Technical and Medical business with Blackwell Publishing.

Registered office
John Wiley & Sons Ltd, The Atrium, Southern Gate, Chichester, West Sussex, PO19 8SQ,
United Kingdom

Editorial office
John Wiley & Sons Ltd, The Atrium, Southern Gate, Chichester, West Sussex, PO19 8SQ,
United Kingdom

For details of our global editorial offices, for customer services and for information about how
to apply for permission to reuse the copyright material in this book please see our website at
www.wiley.com/wiley-blackwell.

Library of Congress Cataloging-in-Publication Data

Central venous catheters/editors, Helen Hamilton, Andrew R. Bodenham.
    p. ; cm.
Includes bibliographical references and index.
ISBN 978-0-470-01994-8 (pbk. alk. paper)   1. Intravenous catheterization.
2. Blood-vessels–Cutdown.   3. Nursing.   I. Hamilton, Helen, 1944-   II. Bodenham, Andrew.
[DNLM: 1. Catheterization, Central Venous. WB 365 C397 2009]
RC683.5.I5C46 2009
617′.05–dc22

                                                                                                    2008027932

A catalogue record for this book is available from the British Library.

Set in 10/12 pt Sabon by Aptara® Inc., New Delhi, India
Printed in Singapore by Markono Print Media Pte Ltd

1   2009

Contents

Contributors

Liz Bishop MSc, BSc (Nurse), RGN, Nurse Consultant, Guys Hospital, London, UK

Andrew R. Bodenham FRCA, Consultant in Anaesthesia and Intensive Care Medicine, Leeds General Infirmary, Leeds, UK

Jonathon Chantler FRCA, MBBChir, MRCP, Consultant Anaesthetic and Intensive Care Consultant, Oxford Radcliffe Hospitals NHS Trust, Headley Way, Headington, Oxford, UK

Sarah Drewett Bsc (hons), CMS, RGN, Clinical Nurse Specialist, Stoke Mandeville Hospital, Aylesbury, Buckinghamshire, UK

T.S.J. Elliott BM, BS, BTech, BMedSci, MRCP, FRCPath, PhD, DSc, Consultant Microbiologist, Director of Acute Medicine, Deputy Medical Director, University Hospital Birmingham NHS Foundation Trust, Selly Oak Hospital, Raddlebarn Road, Selly Oak, Birmingham, UK

Catherine Farrow SpR Anaesthesia, Leeds General Infirmary, Leeds, UK

Janice Gabriel Mphil, PgD, BSc (hons), RN, FETC, ONC, Cert MHS, Nurse Director, Central South Coast Cancer Network, South Central SHA, Oakley Road, Southampton, UK

Simon Galloway FRCA, Consultant in Anaesthesia, Bradford Royal Infirmary, Duckworth Lane, Bradford, UK

Andrew Gratrix FRCA, Consultant in Intensive Care and Anaesthesia, Hull Royal Infirmary, Anlaby Road, Hull, UK

Helen Hamilton CBE, FRCN, RGN, Independent nurse consultant, intravenous therapy, Oxford Radcliffe Hospitals Trust, Oxfordshire, UK

Fiona Ives BSc (hons), RGN, Formerly at the Addenbrooks Hospital, Cambridge, UK

Cathy Hartley-Jones Latterly of Oxford Radcliffe Hospitals NHS Trust, Oxford, UK

Julian Millo BSc, MBBS, MRCP, FRCA, DICM, Consultant Anaesthetist, Oxford, UK

J.L. Peters BSc, FRCS, Consultant General Surgeon, Princess Alexandra Hospital, Harlow, Essex, UK

Jane Phillips-Hughes MBBChir, MRCP, FRCR, Consultant Radiologist, Oxford Radcliffe Hospitals NHS Trust, Headley Way, Headington, Oxford, UK

Liz Simcock BA (hons), RCN, Clinical Nurse Specialist for Central Venous Access, UCL Hospitals NHS Foundation Trust, Haematology/Oncology Daycare, London, UK

Dinuke R. Warakaulle MRCP, FRCR, Consultant Radiologist, Department of Radiology, Stoke Mandeville Hospital, Aylesbury, Buckinghamshire, UK

Nancy Moureau BSN, CRNI, Nurse Consultant, Placement and Management of peripherally inserted catheters, Hartwell, USA

Preface

There has been an explosion of interest in the area of central venous catheterisation with an estimated 250,000 such procedures annually in the UK alone. The traditional use of catheters in anaesthesia, critical care, surgery and acute medicine continues, and there is also a rapidly increasing requirement for medium or longer-term central venous catheterisation for parenteral nutrition, cancer chemotherapy, prolonged antibiotics and other interventions. A wide variety of different professionals are involved with the insertion, care and removal of such devices.

This title was conceived to fill a gap in information related to central venous catheterisation. There is a huge amount of information available from multiple sources often in the form of small case series, case reports, institutional clinical protocols and other anecdotal information, together with an increasing number of randomised controlled trials to guide practice. However, there are relatively few books either in the UK or worldwide covering this topic in any depth. Available books tend to be either rather basic or very specialised, relating to interventional radiology or other disciplines. We have aimed with this publication to provide a reasonably detailed account of most clinical applications of central venous catheters. It is hoped the book will provide useful guidance for both consultants and trainees in medical disciplines and the increasing number of nurses and other professionals involved in this area. Unlike other books, we have tried to give as much emphasis on patient assessment, aftercare and management of catheters as we have on the original insertion procedures. Other issues which are often ignored in other books like removal and infection are also extensively covered.

We thank all our authors and the publishers for their time and commitment in making this book come together and would welcome any feedback from interested readers.

Chapter 1

The history of central venous access

J.L. Peters

Introduction

Techniques and indications for venous access are rapidly changing with huge advances in the last 60 years. An appreciation of such developments and earlier historical endeavours in this field allow the reader insight into the origins of many modern-day practices and the devices in use.

The origins of venous access

Up to the time of William Harvey (1578–1657), there was considerable debate about the circulation. Shortly after Harvey's discovery, Sir Christopher Wren (1971) made the first attempts at providing intravenous nutrition and injecting drugs. In 1656, using a goose quill attached to a pig's bladder, he infused a mixture of wine, ale and opium into dogs. He was not alone in this field of inquiry, for Lower and King (1662), Lower (1932) and Major (1667) performed intravenous infusions and transfusions on animals. Major also used the silver cannula and a pig's bladder to infuse saline via the antecubital fossa veins in a human being. An illustration of this technique can be found in the Wellcome History of Medicine Museum in London. Robert Boyle described the work of Wren, and he performed experiments using intravenous infusion from animals to humans (Birch 1744, Wheatley 1966). Denys (1667) transfused blood from a lamb into a human being in 1667 in Paris, and Lower performed the first successful transfusion of animal blood into a human being in the same year. These practices soon fell into disrepute, as fatal reactions occurred. A church and parliamentary edict prevented further transfusions until 1818, when Blundell (1818), an English obstetrician, saved the lives of several patients with postpartum haemorrhage by injecting blood using a syringe.

In 1733, Stephen Hales conceived the idea of introducing a glass tube into the venous and arterial systems of a live mare in order to measure blood pressure. He also made the first attempts to estimate the cardiac output by bleeding the animal to death and filling its left ventricle with melted beeswax. He multiplied the volume of the solidified wax by the normal resting heart rate in order to achieve figures for the cardiac output of dogs, oxen, sheep and humans (Hales 1974).

Cardiac catheterisation was first performed by Claude Bernard in France to determine the temperature of the blood in the right and left ventricles. Hoff *et al.* (1965) had suggested that animal heat was produced as a result of respiratory gas exchange in the lungs, whilst Magnus (1837) had advanced the alternative hypothesis that 'combustion' took place in the tissues. In 1844, Bernard (1876) operated on a horse and cannulated the carotid artery and left ventricle, followed by the internal jugular vein and right ventricle, using a long mercury thermometer. He disproved the pulmonary combustion theory, and later he went on to measure intracardiac pressures using glass tubes. Bernard (1876) also noted in an autopsy on a dog that the right ventricle had been perforated by the tube, causing intrapericardial haemorrhage, and thus he recorded the first complication of central venous catheterisation. The thrust of these investigations was to try and determine why the living body was warm compared to the coldness of a corpse.

The first systemic study, description and interpretation of intracardiac pressure recordings were made by Chauveau and Marey (1863) after working at the School of Veterinary Medicine of Alfort near Paris. They developed a special double lumen catheter, and Marey wrote:

one can be reassured of the innocuity of this method by examining the horse, who is scarcely disturbed, walks and eats as usual. In only a few instances is the pulse rate slightly increased, especially at the time of the catheter's introduction within the heart cavities.

Thus, he first noted the potential for arrhythmias to occur as a complication of insertion. He also emphasised the importance of extending the clinical examination to include the exploration of many cavities and canalicular systems with catheters; however, neither he nor Chauveau extended their investigations to humans. During the following years cardiac catheterisation developed rapidly as an investigation in circulatory physiology and new manometric systems were developed. Rolleston (1887) pointed out the role of friction along the tube from the exploring cannula to the manometer. Porter (1892) studied the canine heart using silver-plated brass tubes with a single or double lumen and an internal diameter of 3 mm, connected by a 30–40-cm-long rubber tubing with the same diameter as the manometer. At this time, arguments surrounded the question of whether or not such catheters and manometers accurately reflected the intracardiac pressures. These questions were finally resolved by Franck (1903, 1905) when he published his classic papers.

Controversy surrounds the earliest pioneers of central venous catheterisation in humans. Werner Forssmann, André Cournand and Dickinson Richards jointly shared the 1956 Nobel Prize for Medicine. The first to report the use of a catheter in humans for obtaining mixed venous blood for the measurement of right atrial pressure or cardiac output were Cournand and Ranges (1941). They mention Forssmann (1929) as the originator of central venous catheterisation technique. In 1929, shortly after the publication of Forssmann's paper in which he described his self-catheterisation experiment, an addendum was published in which Forssmann referred to a communication stating:

> *Professor E Unger informs me that Bleichroeder, Unger and Loeb carried out the same experiment in 1912. This was published under the title – 'Intra-arterielle Therapie'. He [Unger] had passed a ureteric catheter into the arm veins up to the axilla on four human subjects, among them Dr Bleichroeder, and also from the thigh to the vena cava. To judge from the length of the catheter and a stabbing pain, he believed that in the case of Dr Bleichroeder, the catheter must reach the right heart. This latter experiment was not published.*

The reference provided by Unger alluded to presentations by Bleichroeder, Unger and Loeb (1912) before the Hufeland Medical Society in Berlin. Bleichroeder reported in 1905 that he had passed catheters into the arteries and veins of dogs as well as of human beings. He did not believe the experiments to be of any practical value and left them unpublished. However, in 1912, with the opening of the 'chemotherapeutic era', he perceived a use for his method, as it was believed at the time that a chemotherapeutic agent should be applied as near as possible to the diseased organ. Thus, in four patients with puerperal sepsis, Bleichroeder and Unger inserted a catheter via the femoral artery up to the region of the aortic bifurcation and injected 'collargol'. In his address, Bleichroeder (1904) did not specify the nature of his experiments, but remarked that he had used the catheter to obtain blood from the inferior vena cava close to the hepatic vein. He was interested in the morbid anatomy of cirrhosis, and these investigations may have been related. In his paper concerning intra-arterial therapy, he stated that he had passed the catheter well over a hundred times through the femoral vein and left it in place for several hours without clot formation or other ill-effects. Naturally, he was unable to verify the exact position of catheters using contrast radiology.

Forssmann (1931) conceived the idea of introducing a catheter into the right heart in order to administer emergency drugs on the operating table, in the most rapid and effective way, during episodes of sudden cardiac failure. He was opposed to percutaneous intracardiac injections because of the risks of cardiac tamponade, from either a coronary vessel laceration caused by the needle or leakage of blood from the heart itself, and of pneumothorax from pleural laceration. He first attempted the approach on cadavers using a vein in the antecubital fossa of the left arm. He chose the left arm because the catheter had to make less of a curve when it passed through the subclavian and innominate veins. He also realised that this occurred because of the relatively acute angle at which various tributaries entered the main brachial, axillary and subclavian veins, pointing always in the direction of blood flow.

At the time, Forssmann was working in the small town of Eberswalde, 50 miles northeast of Berlin, as assistant in the surgical department under Dr Schneider. Although a friend and mentor, Schneider denied permission for Forssmann's plans to attempt the procedure on patients or on himself. Forssmann could not be deterred, however, and he decided to carry out the experiment upon himself. A wide-bore needle was inserted into a right cubital fossa vein, through which a ureteric catheter (4 French) was passed for 35 cm without difficulty. His colleague, who performed the operation, flinched and abandoned the procedure. One week later, Forssmann anaesthetised his own left cubital fossa, advanced the catheter into his right atrium and then climbed several flights of stairs to the X-ray department and documented his achievement. This account was published on 5 November 1929. The first and only clinical application in which he used his catheter was to administer glucose, epinephrine hydrochloride and strophanthin to a woman with terminal purulent peritonitis following perforation of the appendix. After a temporary improvement, the patient relapsed and died; at autopsy, the catheter was found to have passed through the right atrium and its tip was situated in the inferior vena cava.

Forssmann (1931) pointed out that such a catheter could be used for central venous blood sampling as well as for injections. He also realised that the technique he had pioneered provided many possibilities for future metabolic studies and investigations into cardiac function. Later he was the first to inject a radio-opaque substance directly into the right heart via both arm and thigh veins (on himself) using uroselectan. Thus, he demonstrated that a well-known experimental technique could be applied to the study and treatment of disease in humans.

His enthusiasm for this discovery did not extend to his contemporary German colleagues, and little interest was shown in his work. He spent 6 years as an army surgeon in Germany, Norway and Russia and returned weary and malnourished to civilian medical practice. He turned to urology before receiving his unexpected and belated academic reward.

A short hiatus in this field of clinical physiology occurred until the systemic physiological investigations of Cournand, Richards and others commenced in 1936. A new flexible radio-opaque catheter was designed to enable intravenous and intracardiac blood sampling to be performed together with pressure recordings in the right atrium and pulmonary artery. They performed studies in heart failure, valvular heart disease and shock, and stimulated many other workers in this field around the world. For those who may be particularly interested, a definitive account of this period has been provided by Cournand (1975).

The introduction of flexible polyethylene cannulas for intravenous feeding in children was introduced by Meyers (1945) and Zimmerman (1945), and this innovation from the plastics industry heralded the beginning of an era in intravenous therapy and diagnostic intervention. Surgeons adapted the tubing with ingenuity; for example, the palliative treatment of obstructive hydrocephalus became a reality in May 1949, when Nulsen and Spitz (1952) established a valved shunt between the right lateral ventricle and the right internal jugular vein. They recognised the failure of the intravascular prosthesis caused by thrombosis inside the shunt and the jugular vein. The techniques derived from this procedure are now applicable for the direct cannulation of the internal jugular vein in the most difficult cases requiring parenteral nutrition.

The mass production of cannulas and central catheters consisting of polyvinyl chloride was inevitably followed by numerous clinical case reports and series describing local and systemic complications (Morris 1955, Moncrief 1958, Crane 1960, Doering *et al.* 1967, Neuhof and Seley 1974). Indar (1959) pointed out the problem of thrombosis which occurred when polyethylene catheters were used in the deep veins. Industry thus continued to research for improved inert materials for use as intravascular prostheses. Tetrafluoroethylene (TFE) and fluoroethylenepolypropylene (FEP) have been used and the incidence of thrombosis reduced as a result.

Quinton *et al.* (1960) jointly developed a Teflon and subsequently a Silastic arteriovenous shunt for use in haemodialysis. This advance has proved to be of tremendous significance in the achievement of safe chronic venous access. A Silastic intravenous catheter was introduced (Stewart and Sanislow 1961) at Ann Arbor Hospital, Michigan. The tubing they used was extruded and cured at 480°F for 16 hours, the cannula being connected to the intravenous administration set by a 20-gauge needle after the point had been removed by grinding. Herein lies a problem of the inertness of silicone; namely, it is extremely difficult to bond the catheter to the hub securely. Mechanical catheter-related problems have now assumed importance in the care of patients receiving prolonged intravenous therapy (Fleming *et al.* 1980). Design alterations are still needed in order to make further improvements in this aspect of patient care.

Current central venous access devices are fabricated from silicone, polyurethane or polyamide and research continues to provide reduced thrombogenicity of the intravascular portion of the device and at the same time provide a strengthened durability of the extravascular and extracorporeal segment of the infusion system.

Venous access and the development of parenteral nutrition

During the past 30 years, there has been a substantial increase in the number of patients who have received parenteral nutritional support in hospital. The terminology emerging from the scientific literature includes such new abbreviations as IVH (intravenous hyperalimentation) and TPN (total parenteral nutrition). Following the refinement of long-life silicone tunnelled catheters introduced by Scribner *et al.* (1970) and Broviac *et al.* (1973), home parenteral nutrition (HPN) has emerged as a reality for a few carefully selected patients. The infusion of energy substrates and nitrogen has been established as an integral feature of the supportive medical care of patients during severe medical or surgical illness.

The progress from the experiments by Sir Christopher Wren in 1656, when he infused wine, ale and opium into dogs, follows a fascinating path. John Hunter made some poignant observations throughout his surgical career; in his *Treatise on the Blood, Inflammation and Gun-Shot Wounds* published in 1794, Hunter discussed the aspect of wound healing which he termed 'union by the first intention'. The words he used then and which have often been quoted since are:

> *It will be proper to observe here that there is a circumstance attending accidental injury which does not belong to the disease, viz. that the injury done, has in all cases a tendency to produce both the disposition and means of cure.* (Hunter 1794)

Central venous catheters have played a vital role in current medical and surgical practice enabling clinicians to monitor, augment and support the efforts of the body to stabilise the circulation during (or following) major surgery and provide nutritional supplements in order to fire the 'disposition and means of cure'.

Following its isolation and purification, glucose was used intravenously in animals by Bernard (1843). Latta (1831) administered an infusion of water and saline to an elderly victim of cholera. Six pints were given intravenously in 6 minutes and the first complication of intravenous therapy recorded – circulatory overload. The populations of Asia, Europe and North America were intermittently attacked by epidemics of cholera and typhoid throughout the eighteenth century, and some of the earliest crude attempts at providing fluids and nutrition were made on the unfortunate victims of this disease.

In 1859, Hodder (1873) of Toronto suggested to his friend James Bovell that it would be 'proper and a probable success' to transfuse blood into cholera victims. Bovell pointed out that the supply would quickly run out in an epidemic as few people would be willing to part with their blood, and they could not be sure the blood itself would not be diseased. This is the first record of infusion contamination being contemplated as a hazard. Hodder felt that the nearest available analogue of blood in abundant supply was milk, and he knew that it had been given intravenously to animals by Donné without a fatal result. Hodder and Bovell bided their time, and in 1873, the city fathers of Toronto were just as unprepared for cholera as in 1859. An old shed in the hospital grounds was made ready and the first cholera victim brought in a state of circulatory collapse. Four other medical officers were consulted and agreed about the diagnosis and hopeless prognosis. On announcing his planned experiment, Hodder was told he would kill the patient. All but one of the medical officers refused to stay and observe the proceedings. A cow was brought to the shed, milked into a bowl, the milk was filtered through a gauze and 14 ounces injected through a tube inserted in a cut-down venesection from a warmed syringe. The effect was 'magical' and the patient recovered his pulse and survived. Two other patients had this form of treatment, rallied and died during Hodder's absence from the shed. Hodder and Bovell were the first to realise that the cost of the nutritional fluids and apparatus could be a limiting factor in the provision of their treatment. They applied to the corporation for a cow and a few items 'indispensably necessary for the comfort and well being of patients'; these were refused and they thereupon sent in their resignation!

Malcolm (1893) published a classic description of *The Physiology of Death from Traumatic Fever* and noted that shock was simply one of the phenomena caused by injury, whether surgical or otherwise, rather than a complication. His work stimulated the study of metabolic processes in shock. The value of glucose infusions for patients was not accepted immediately. The work of Pasteur and Joubert (1877) had provided the impetus to produce sterile solutions for animal and clinical use. Sugar was first infused in humans by Briedl and Kraus (1971) in 1896, and Kausch (1911) first infused glucose for postoperative nutritional purposes in 1911.

The concept of providing intravenous nutrition was furthered when, in 1913, Henriques and Andersen (1961) injected protein hydrolysate, glucose and salt solution into goats for 16 days. Murlin and Ritchie (1916) infused fat experimentally for the first time in 1916, and 4 years later, Yamakawa (1920) was the first to use an intravenous infusion of fat in humans. The significance of this early work was overlooked until 1937 when Elman and his colleagues performed their experiments. Several basic questions concerning the metabolic response to injury were being investigated by Sir David Cuthbertson during the 1930s. He made a teleological proposition (Cuthbertson 1929, 1930) that an injured animal in response to injury is faced with a diminished food supply, and he suggested that the rapid early catabolism of tissues could be associated with the first signs of regeneration of the injured part. Cuthbertson (1929–1931) went on to perform outstanding investigations into many aspects of the catabolic response to injury. Cuthbertson (1936) pointed out that a high-protein and high-calorie diet after fractures of the long bones was beneficial in attenuating the marked loss of body proteins. Cuthbertson (1942) introduced the terms 'ebb phase' and 'flow phase' for the initial depressed period of metabolism and the later period of increased metabolic rate after trauma.

Elman (1937) demonstrated the effectiveness of a 5% amino acid mixture derived from a sulphuric acid hydrolysate of casein to which tryptophan and cystine were added. In dogs depleted of their blood by acute haemorrhage, regeneration of the plasma proteins was evident after 6 hours in the group fed with 5% amino acid and 5% glucose, whilst the controls who were given 10% glucose showed no evidence of plasma protein repletion after 6 hours and very little after 24 hours. Elman and Weiner (1939) reported the first use of protein hydrolysate in humans. Positive nitrogen balance was maintained in postoperative patients and in patients with inoperable carcinoma by providing 20 g of casein hydrolysate, tryptophan supplement, glucose and saline. Shol and Blackfan (1940) described the first artificial amino acid mixture used intravenously in humans.

During World War II, the importance of this work was becoming apparent. It was recognised that intravenous therapy with protein hydrolysates and 5 or 10% glucose given through peripheral veins failed to provide sufficient non-protein calories to ensure that administered amino acids would be used for tissue protein synthesis and regeneration rather than for immediate energy purposes. The alternatives were to give large volumes of fluid or very concentrated solutions. Fat emulsions were a promising alternative source of energy. The observation that the body could tolerate the intravenous fat emulsion issuing from the thoracic duct provided the proof which stimulated Wretlind to search for a suitable alternative emulsion that could be manufactured. In the USA, an emulsion derived from cottonseed oil (Lipomul) was associated with toxic reactions, and all fat emulsions were removed from the market. Wretlind and his co-workers in Sweden embarked upon a long series of experiments using an animal test system to find a suitable emulsion. Hakasson (1968) finally developed a soybean oil and egg yolk phospholipid emulsion free of toxic reactions, and the experimental dogs survived the 28-day test period. A study performed by Hallberg *et al.* (1966) found that patients were able to tolerate this compound (Intralipid), and in 1965, an adult patient with Crohn's disease was kept in a good nutritional state for 5 months, fed intravenously with amino acids, glucose, fat, electrolytes and vitamins. In the UK, Rickham (1967) and his colleagues started to use intravenous fat emulsions together with amino acids and sugar solutions in paediatric surgical practice during the period 1962–1967 for children who had required extensive intestinal resection. Hadfield (1966) administered high-calorie intravenous feeding in surgical patients whilst he was at the Radcliffe Infirmary, Oxford. He used Intralipid in combination with casein hydrolysates and noted reductions in the postoperative weight loss of patients undergoing partial gastrectomy and also improvements in the serum protein levels of patients with ulcerative colitis and severe intestinal malabsorption.

At the same time as these advances were being made in Stockholm and the UK, the use of concentrated glucose as an alternative energy source was being investigated in the USA. Following careful fundamental research into the metabolic care of surgical patients, Francis Moore (1959) in Boston described the use of the superior vena cava for the infusion of concentrated glucose. He also stated that 'patients on prolonged intravenous feeding rarely gain weight by tissue synthesis, yet it is conceivable that this might some day occur as intravenous hyperalimentation is perfected and concentrated'. Dudrick *et al.* (1966) reported that they could successfully perform total parenteral nutrition in beagle dogs and match orally fed controls in weight gain, development and growth. Dudrick *et al.* (1967, 1968) and Wilmore and Dudrick (1968) went on to report similar results in humans. They were able to achieve their remarkable results in free-moving beagle puppies by using fine catheters, which after insertion into the central veins were tunnelled subcutaneously for a distance to the back of the animal's neck. Such catheters were kept in place for periods of 72–256 days of intravenous hyperalimentation. The American investigators used concentrated glucose solutions in order to provide an adequate calorific intake, and for this to be accomplished without a high incidence of thrombosis or phlebitis, a central venous infusion system was developed. This would appear to be the first recognition of the beneficial effects of tunnelling catheters and coincided with the development of the Hickman and Broviac catheters on the West Coast of the USA.

The need to provide an adequate supply of protein, calories, vitamins and trace elements to patients undergoing major surgery, following severe trauma or recuperating from intercurrent disease is well recognised. Peaston (1968) summarised the situation succinctly by stating:

> *In recent years, materials have become available whereby intravenous nutrition can be adequately maintained. The therapeutic decision not to use them is a positive action to starve the patient, and must in itself be justified unless the complications from their use outweigh the advantages conferred.*

Johnston (1979) suggests that when nutritional support has to be provided by the intravenous route, as much as 1600 calories may be provided per day in an adult by peripheral venous infusion. This should be the route of choice in patients requiring short-term nutritional support. However, where prolonged therapy is required, the incidence of painful thrombophlebitis becomes unacceptable for most patients and central catheterisation must be employed. The biochemistry and methodology of providing supplementary or total parenteral nutrition has steadily progressed and several comprehensive reviews have been produced (Bernard 1971).

Venous access and chemotherapy

This has been referred to previously in the initial historical development of this technique. The origins of peripherally inserted central catheters (PICCs) obviously can be attributed to Werner Forssmann. The advent of effective anti-cancer treatment for a variety of tumours which required prolonged venous access and multiple, often daily peripheral blood sampling, led to the development and introduction in 1975, by Hickman *et al.* (1979), of the Hickman Silastic catheter, which possessed a 1.6-mm lumen and a Dacron cuff, for prolonged intravenous therapy in patients with leukaemia and allied disorders. This has proved to be an invaluable innovation for the comfort and care of patients with such severe disorders. It was shown that the incidence of septicaemia, in patients having both their blood samples removed and receiving their intravenous fluids, chemotherapy and haematological support by the solitary Hickman catheter, was less than in the control group of patients being managed with conventional peripheral intravenous therapy (Hickman *et al.* 1979). A similar experience was also reported from The Royal Marsden Hospital, London, by Thomas (1979), and Blacklock *et al.*

(1980) and colleagues working in Auckland, New Zealand. The Broviac catheter was of similar design with a finer lumen for the infusion of parenteral nutrition. These catheter types have evolved into multi-lumen variants. Modifications have been made to the tip, e.g. the Groshong catheter, in an effort to prevent reflux of blood into the lumen of the catheter resulting in the formation of thrombus, or influx of air due to a negative venous pressure.

Routes of insertion

The percutaneous internal jugular approach was developed by Dr Ian English *et al.* in 1968 for central venous pressure monitoring and intra-operative and post-operative fluid infusion at The Brompton Hospital, London (English *et al.* 1969a, b). Branthwaite and Bradley (1968) reported the use of the Seldinger technique to introduce fine-bore cannulas fitted with thermistors via the internal jugular vein, whilst they investigated the measurement of cardiac output using the thermodilution principle at St Thomas Hospital, London. Other descriptions and variations of surgical technique were subsequently published (Boulanger *et al.* 1976, Prince *et al.* 1976, Rao *et al.* 1977, Coté *et al.* 1979).

Percutaneous infraclavicular subclavian vein catheterisation

The veins of the arm were used exclusively for central venous cannulation, when Aubaniac (1952) first introduced the concept of using the infraclavicular subclavian vein as a site for venepuncture. His technique was adopted by Keeri-Szanto (1956), Villafane (1953) and Lepp (1953). Initially, the technique was restricted to venepuncture for obtaining blood samples or giving injections, and central catheterisation via the subclavian vein was not performed. In 1954, Aubaniac performed angiocardiography using this approach. A further 8 years elapsed before Wilson *et al.* (1962) pioneered the introduction of flexible central catheters into the superior vena cava by this route. The technique was first described in the UK by Ashbaugh and Thompson (1963), while they were working in Edinburgh.

A supraclavicular approach to subclavian vein catheterisation

The introduction of cannulas into the subclavian vein via percutaneous techniques found favour by those clinicians who thought this might be a way of avoiding the complication of pneumothorax. Yoffa (1965) introduced the percutaneous supraclavicular approach to the subclavian vein for this reason. Argument continues as to whether the supraclavicular or the infraclavicular approach is safer.

Imaging

The development of techniques to carefully check the intravascular site of the catheter, e.g. X-ray imaging, are, of course, not new but were introduced by Forssmann at the very outset. It has also taken some time for the use of ultrasound to be adopted for safer placement of central venous catheters. The author and his colleagues (Peters *et al.* 1982) used this technique in the late 1970s at University College Hospital, London. The continuing search for safer techniques must be pursued in order to avoid unnecessary and often catastrophic complications.

Conclusion

This chapter, hopefully, will provide a historical foundation for this manual and will indicate the needs and opportunities for improvements in this field of clinical practice.

References

Ashbaugh D, Thompson JW (1963). Subclavian vein infusion. *Lancet* 2:1138.

Aubaniac R (1952). L'injection intraveneuse sous claviculaire. *Presse Médicale.* 60:1456.

Bernard C (1876). *Leçons sur la Chaleur Animale.* Librairie J.-B. Baillière et Fils, Paris, pp. 42–81.

Bernard C (1971). New horizons for intravenous feeding. *JAMA* 215:939–949.

Birch T (ed.) (1744). *The Works of the Honourable Robert Boyle in Five Volumes.* Millar, London, UK.

Blacklock HA, Hill RS, Clarke AG et al. (1980). Use of a modified subcutaneous right atrial catheter for venous access in leukaemic patients. *Lancet* 1:993.

Bleichroeder F (1904). *Virch. Arch. Pathol.* 177:435.

Bleichroeder F (1912). *Berl. Klin. Wochenschr.* 49:1503.

Blundell J (1818). *Medico-Chirur. Trans.* 9:56–92.

Boulanger M, Delva E, Maille JG et al. (1976). Internal jugular vein cannulation. *Canadian Anaesthetists Society Journal* 123:609–615.

Branthwaite MA, Bradley RD (1968). Measurement of cardiac output by thermal dilution in man. *Journal of Applied Physiology* 24:434–438.

Briedl A, Kraus R (1971). New horizons for intravenous feeding. *JAMA* 215:939–949.

Broviac JW, Cole JJ, Scribner BH (1973). A silicone rubber atrial catheter for prolonged parenteral alimentation. *Surgery, Gynecology and Obstetrics* 136:602–606.

Chauveau A, Marey EJ (1863). Appareils et Expériences Cardiographiques. Demonstration Nouvelle du Mécanisme des Mouvements du Coeur par l'emploi des Instruments Enregistreurs à Indications Continués. *Mem. Acad. Médé.* 26:268.

Coté CJ, Jobes DR, Schwartz AJ et al. (1979). Two approaches to cannulation of a child's internal jugular vein. *Anaesthesiology* 50:371–373.

Cournand A (1975). Cardiac catheterisation. Development of the technique, its contributions to experimental medicine, and its initial application in man. *Acta Medica Scandinavica* 579(Suppl):7–32.

Cournand A, Ranges HA (1941). Catheterisation of the right auricle in man. *Proceedings of the Society for Experimental Biology and Medicine* 46:462.

Crane C (1960). Venous interruption for septic thrombophlebitis. *New England Journal of Medicine* 262:947–951.

Cuthbertson DP (1929). The influence of prolonged muscular rest on metabolism. *Biochemical Journal* 23:1328–1345.

Cuthbertson DP (1930). The disturbance of metabolism produced by bony and non-bony injury, with notes on certain abnormal conditions of bone. *Biochemical Journal* 24:1244–1263.

Cuthbertson DP (1931). The distribution of nitrogen and sulphur in the urine during conditions of increased catabolism. *Biochemical Journal* 25:236–244.

Cuthbertson DP (1936). Further observations on the disturbance of metabolism caused by injury with particular reference to the dietary requirements of fracture cases. *British Journal of Surgery* 23:505–520.

Cuthbertson DP (1942). Post-shock metabolic response. *Lancet* 1:433–437.

Denys JB (1667). *Lettres Touchant Deux Experiences de la Transfusions Fites sur des Hommes*. Cusson, Paris, pp.12–13.

Doering RB, Stemmer EA, Connelly JE (1967). Complications of indwelling venous catheters. *American Journal of Surgery* 114:259–266.

Dudrick SJ, Vars HM, Rhoads JE (1966). Growth of puppies receiving all nutritional requirements by vein. *Fortsch. Parenteral Ernahrung.* 2:16–18.

Dudrick SJ, Wilmore DW, Vars HM (1967). Long-term total parenteral nutrition with growth in puppies and positive nitrogen balance in patients. *Surgical Forum* 18:356–357.

Dudrick SJ, Wilmore DW, Vars HM *et al.* (1968). Long-term parenteral nutrition with growth, development and positive nitrogen balance. *Surgery* 64:134–142.

Elman R (1937): Intravenous injection of amino acids in regeneration of serum protein following severe experimental haemorrhage. *Proceedings of the Society for Experimental Biology and Medicine* 1937; 36:867–870.

Elman R, Weiner DO (1939): Intravenous alimentation with special reference to protein (amino acid) metabolism. *JAMA* 112:796–802.

English IC, Frew RM, Piggott JF, Zaki M (1969a). Percutaneous cannulation of the internal jugular vein. *Anaesthesia* 24:521–531.

English IC, Frew RM, Piggott JF, Zaki M (1969b). Percutaneous cannulation of the internal jugular vein. *Thorax* 24:496–497.

Fleming CR, Witzke DJ, Beart RW (1980). Catheter-related complications in patients receiving home parenteral nutrition. *Annals of Surgery* 192:593–599.

Forssmann W (1929). Die Sondierung des Rechten Herzens. *Klinische Wochenschrift* 8:2085.

Forssmann W (1931). Über Kontrastderstellung der Hohlen des Pebenden rechten Herzens und der lungenschlagadr. *Münchener medizinische Wochenschrift* 78:489–492.

Franck O (1903). Kritik der Elastischen Manometer. *Zeitschrift für Biologie* 44:445.

Franck O (1905). Die Puls in den Arterien. *Zeitschrift für Biologie* 45:441.

Hadfield J (1966). High caloric intravenous feeding in surgical patients. *Clinical Medicine* 73:25–30.

Hakasson I (1968). Experiences in long-term studies on nine fat emulsions in dogs. *Nutritio et Dieta* 10:54–76.

Hales S (1974). Experiment 3. Statistical essays: containing haemastaticks. In *Heart Disease*, White PD (ed.), 3rd edn. Macmillan, New York, p. 92.

Hallberg D, Schuberth O, Wretlind A (1966). Experimental and clinical studies with fat emulsion for intravenous nutrition. *Nutritio et Dieta* 8:245–281.

Henriques V, Andersen AC (1961). *Chemistry of Amino Acids*, Vol. I. Wiley, New York p. 332.

Hickman RO, Buckner CD, Clift R *et al.* (1979). A modified right atrial catheter for access to the venous system in marrow transplant recipients. *Surgery, Gynecology and Obstetrics* 148:871–875.

Hodder EM (1873). Transfusion of milk in cholera. *Practitioner* 10:14–16.

Hoff HE, Guillemin R, Sakiz E (1965). Claude Bernard on animal heat. An unpublished manuscript and some original notes. *Perspectives in Biology and Medicine* 7:347–368.

Hunter J (1794). *A Treatise on Blood Information and Gunshot Wounds*. Nicol, London, UK.

Indar R (1959). The dangers of indwelling polyethylene catheters in deep veins. *Lancet* 1:284–286.

Johnston IDA (1979). Parenteral nutrition in the cancer patient. *Journal of Human Nutrition* 33:189–196.

Kausch W (1911). Über intravenose and subcutane Ernahrung mit Traubenzucker. *Deutsche Medizinische Wochenschrift* 37:8–9.

Keeri-Szanto M (1956). The subclavian vein: a constant and convenient intravenous injection site. *Archives of Surgery* 72:179.

Latta T (1831). Injections of saline solution in extraordinary quantities into the veins of cases of malignant cholera (Letter). *Lancet* 2:243.

Lepp H (1953). On a new intravenous injection and puncture method; infraclavicular puncture of the subclavian vein (translation). *Deutsche zahnärztliche Zeitschrift* 8:511–512.

Lower R (1932). Tractatus de Corde, 1669. In *Early Science in Oxford*, Vol. IX, Franklin KJ (trans.). Oxford Press, London, UK.

Lower R, King E (1662). An account of the experiment of transfusion. *Philosophical Transaction* 2:557–564.

Magnus G (1837). Über die im Blute enthaltenen Gase. Sauerstoffe, Stickstoff und Kohlensäure. *Ann. Phys. Chem.* 12:583.

Major JD (1667). *Chirurgia Infusorii.* Reumannus, Kilonia, Germany.

Malcolm JD (1893). *The Physiology of Death from Traumatic Fever.* Churchill, London, UK.

Meyers L (1945). Intravenous catheterisation. *American Journal of Nursing* 45:930–931.

Moncrief JA (1958). Femoral catheters. *Annals of Surgery* 147:166–172.

Moore FD (1959). *Metabolic Care of the Surgical Patient.* WB Saunders, Philadelphia, PA, pp.25–48, 49–68.

Morris J (1955). Thrombophlebitis following intravenous infusions. *Lancet* 1:154

Murlin JR, Ritchie JA (1916). The fat of the blood in relation to heat production, narcosis and muscular work. *American Journal of Physiology* 40:146.

Neuhof H, Seley GP (1974). Acute suppurative phlebitis complicated by septicaemia. *Surgery* 21:831–842.

Nulsen F, Spitz EB (1952). Treatment of hydrocephalus by direct shunt from ventricle to jugular vein. In *Proceedings of 37th Clinical Congress of the American College of Surgeons*, San Francisco, CA. *Surgery Forum*, 399–403.

Pasteur L, Joubert JF (1877). Charbon and septicémie. *Comptes Rendus Hebdomadaires des Séances de l'Académie des Sciences Paris* 85:101–115.

Peaston MJT (1968). Parenteral nutrition in serious illness. *British Journal of Hospital Medicine* 1:708–711.

Peters JL, Belsham P, Garrett CPO *et al.* (1982). Doppler ultrasound an aid to percutaneous infraclavicular subclavian vein catheterisation. *American Journal of Surgery* 143(3):391–393.

Porter WT (1892). Researches in the filling of the heart. *Journal of Physiology* 13:513.

Prince SR, Sullivan RL, Hackel A (1976). Percutaneous catheterisation of the internal jugular vein in infants and children. *Anaesthesiology* 44:170–174.

Quinton WE, Dillard DH, Scribner BH (1960). Cannulation of blood vessels for prolonged haemodialysis. *Transaction of American Society Artificial Internal Organs* 6:104, 1962; 8:236.

Rao TLK, Wong AY, Salem MR (1977). A new approach to percutaneous catheterisation of the internal jugular vein. *Anaesthesiology* 46:362–364.

Rickham PP (1967). Massive small bowel resection in new-born infants. *Annals of the Royal College of Surgeons of England* 41:480–492.

Rolleston HD (1887). Observations on the endocardial pressure curve. *Journal of Physiology* 8:235.

Scribner BH, Cole JJ, Christopher G (1970). Long term total parenteral nutrition: the concept of an artificial gut. *JAMA* 212:457–463.

Shol AT, Blackfan KD (1940). The intravenous administration of crystalline amino acids to infants. *Journal of Nutrition* 20:305–316.

Stewart RD, Sanislow CA (1961). Silastic intravenous catheter. *New England Journal of Medicine* 265:1283–1285.

Thomas M (1979). The use of the Hickman catheter in the management of patients with leukaemia and other malignancies. *British Journal of Surgery* 66:673–674.

Villafane EP (1953). Technica de la transfusion por via subclavicular. *Prensa Medica Argentina* 40:2379.

Wheatley HB (1966). *The Diary of Samuel Pepys*, Vol. II. Random House, New York.

Wilmore DW, Dudrick SJ (1968). Growth and development of an infant receiving all nutrients exclusively by vein. *JAMA* 203:140–144.

Wilson JN, Grown JB, Demong CV *et al.* (1962). Central venous pressure in optimal blood volume maintenance. *Archives of Surgery* 85:563.

Wren C (1971). New horizons for intravenous feeding. *JAMA* 215:939–949.

Yamakawa S (1920). Parenteral nutrition. *Nippon Naika Gakkai Zasshi* 17:122.

Yoffa D (1965). Supraclavicular subclavian venepuncture catheterisation. *Lancet* 2:614–615.

Zimmerman B (1945). Intravenous tubing for parenteral therapy. *Science* 101:566–568.

Chapter 2

Applied anatomy of the central veins

Jonathan Chantler

Introduction

There are at least 250 named veins in the human body. It is probable that all these will have been cannulated at least at some point in history, even if only in error.

Most large vascular structures cannot be visualised externally with the naked eye during cannulation. Furthermore, all central catheters will at some point pass into the great veins of the thorax and abdomen during insertion, where they will follow the course of least resistance, sometimes leading to malposition. It is for these reasons that knowledge of the normal anatomy and common variations is an important component of clinical practice.

What is a central vein?

A central vein is one near the centre of the circulation – the heart. Access to a central vein is required for

- central venous pressure monitoring,
- aspiration of blood,
- large volume fluid infusion,
- infusion of sclerosant drugs and
- right heart catheterisation.

The risk of vein damage from sclerosant infusions is related to the width of the vein and the speed of blood flow down it, rather than its proximity to the heart. In general, the more central the vein, the bigger the vessel and the greater its blood flow. This is most pronounced when the venous system combines into only two vessels, the inferior (IVC) and superior vena cava (SVC), which between them carry virtually the entire cardiac output, approximately 5 L/min at rest in an adult (85 mL/s).

For central venous pressure monitoring, the catheter tip needs to lie beyond the last valve in the vein of access. The most proximal valves to the heart are reliably located in the proximal subclavian, internal jugular and femoral veins. Such valves can easily be visualised with ultrasound scanning.

Veins that satisfy the criteria of being 'big with fast-flowing blood' are the SVC, the brachiocephalic veins, the subclavian veins, the IVC, the external and common iliac veins. Although not a vein as such, the right atrium also satisfies these criteria and can be a suitable place for a central vein catheter tip to lie in some circumstances.

Anatomy of the SVC

The SVC drains venous blood from the upper half of the body. It is formed from the confluence of the two brachiocephalic veins behind the lower border of the first right costal cartilage (Figure 2.1). It is approximately 2 cm wide and has no valves. It is about 7 cm long in the normal adult and descends essentially vertically along a straight path to end in the upper part of the right atrium (Figures 2.2a and 2.2b). It is partly covered

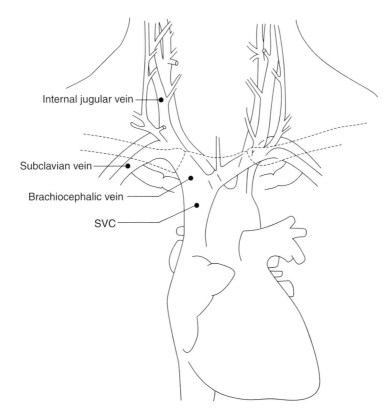

Internal jugular vein

Subclavian vein

Brachiocephalic vein

SVC

Figure 2.1 Diagram of the veins of the neck and chest. The internal jugular veins are seen joining the subclavian veins to form the brachiocephalic or innominate veins. The SVC is formed by the confluence of the brachiocephalic or innominate veins. (Reproduced with permission from John Wiley & Sons, Tortora principles of human anatomy.)

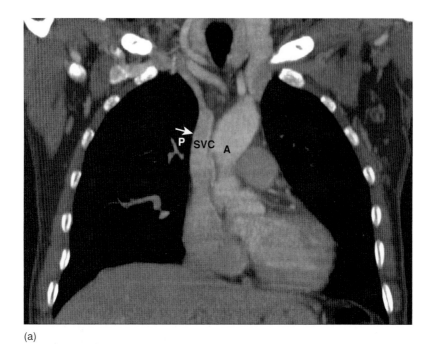

(a)

(b)

Figure 2.2 CT image with contrast showing the anatomy of the SVC. Note the close proximity of SVC, pleura P, the lung, and ascending aorta (A). (a) Coronal section and (b) axial section at level of the pulmonary arteries (PA).

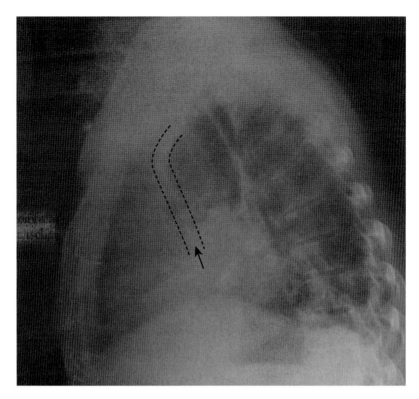

Figure 2.3 Lateral chest X-ray showing central path of a Hickman catheter in the SVC. The dotted lines mark the course of the catheter and the arrow marks its tip.

anteriorly by the right edge of the sternum. In theory, the shadow of its lateral border is visible in anterior–posterior chest X-rays to the right of the sternum, although in practice this is difficult to see. Misplaced catheters lying in the pleura at this site cannot be distinguished from those within the SVC on a plain chest X-ray (see Chapter 12).

As the sternum slopes down anteriorly, the SVC becomes progressively deeper to the skin before ending in the right atrium (Figure 2.3), behind the third right costal cartilage. Its upper right border bulges into the right pleural space with the result that a tear of the vessel in this area risks major haemorrhage into the low-pressure pleural space to cause a haemothorax. This serious complication can be caused from dilators or catheters during insertion. Equally in the longer term, catheter tips (particularly from the left side) can perforate the vein wall and cause a hydrothorax when fluids are infused down the catheter. The ascending aorta lies closely to its left, and misplaced catheters in this part of the aorta may be mistaken to be in the SVC on chest X-ray (see Chapter 12).

The lower half of the vessel is within the fibrous pericardium, which it pierces at the level of the second costal cartilage. This has relevance to the functional anatomy of where the tip of a catheter should lie (see below).

An important major branch of the SVC is the azygos vein, which ascends on the right side in the posterior mediastinum, before arching forward to pierce the posterior wall of the SVC at the level of the fourth thoracic vertebra (Figure 2.4). This junction is about

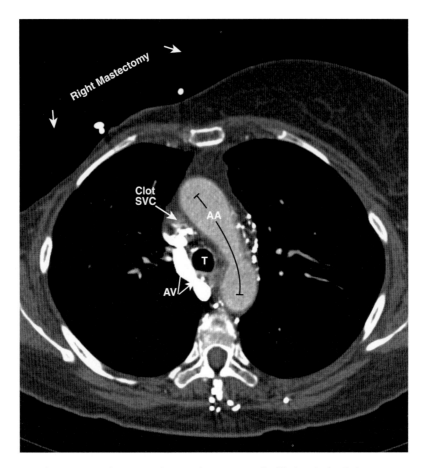

Figure 2.4 Axial CT image with contrast showing the SVC partially filled with clot (lighter appearance compared to patent vein full of X-ray contrast medium) arrow. This clot, which followed long-term venous access, gave rise to a swollen face and arms typical of SVC obstruction. The azygous vein (AV) is seen ascending adjacent to the pleura from posteriorly to join the SVC. Also note the arch of aorta (AA), trachea (T) and site of right mastectomy.

halfway along the SVC and just above the pericardial reflection. The tip of a catheter can potentially lies in this junction or the azygous vein with detrimental consequences.

Anatomy of the IVC

The IVC drains blood from the lower half of the body and is about 2.5 cm wide in the normal adult (Figure 2.1). It is formed by junction of the two common iliac veins and ascends in front of the vertebral column to the right of the aorta. It receives the major renal and hepatic venous systems before piercing the diaphragm and inclining slightly forwards and medially. There are multiple other smaller branches. The intra-thoracic part of the IVC is very short. It soon passes into the pericardium and ascends further to open into the lower posterior part of the right atrium. Within the atrium, there is a valve ('the valve of the IVC') that is largely rudimentary in the adult, but is large and functionally important in the foetus. There are no valves in the IVC itself.

Routes of access to a central vein

The IVC and SVC are generally too difficult to cannulate directly, unless imaging is used, because they lie deeply protected within the chest and abdomen. Therefore, they are usually cannulated more peripherally ('upstream') and a long catheter is passed in the direction of blood flow, often with the help of a guidewire. For instance, the SVC can be reached by cannulating the basilic vein in the antecubital fossa. As the guidewire or catheter advances, it passes in turn through the brachial, axillary, subclavian and brachiocephalic veins before entering the SVC. Similarly, the IVC is reached by cannulation of the femoral vein and the device passes through the external iliac and common iliac veins.

Nine veins are commonly cannulated for percutaneous central venous access. More commonly used veins include

- Subclavian
- Internal jugular
- Femoral
- Basilic (antecubital fossa approach)

Veins used less commonly include

- Axillary (anterior or lateral approaches)
- External jugular
- Brachial (mid upper arm approach)
- Cephalic (antecubital fossa approach)
- Brachiocepahlic (supra-clavicular approach)

In practice, any vein will eventually lead to the heart and given suitable equipment, screening and expertise a small bore catheter could be passed centrally.

Anatomical variations of central veins

These can be congenital or acquired. The high rate of variability is a strong argument for the routine use of imaging techniques for both initial access (if the vein cannot be seen by the naked eye) and subsequent central guidewire and catheter positioning.

Congenital

The commonest variant in the SVC is the so-called left SVC or persistent left SVC. This may occur with or without the normal right SVC. The left SVC is a persistence of the left cardinal vein present in the early foetal circulation that normally atrophies in the adult. The right cardinal vein becomes the right-sided SVC. The right vein (if present) takes the normal course of the SVC. The left crosses the left side of the arch of the aorta, passes in front of the left pulmonary hilum and passes posteriorly to enter the right atrium from behind. Its proximal segment is functionally an enlarged coronary sinus. This vein may communicate with the upper right SVC via a small branch. Its incidence is reported at 1.3% (see Figure 10.1). A left-sided SVC can be used for access, but care should be taken as there are reports of occasional cases where the vein opens into the left atrium with the risk of air or particulate embolism from central catheters (Ghadiali *et al.* 2006).

Below the diaphragm, the IVC can show numerous variations. These are due to abnormalities in the development of the vessels in the foetus. The IVC is normally formed from a dual bilateral circulation (posterior cardinal and sub-cardinal veins), which develops into a single large vessel through right-sided enlargement and left-sided regression. In the adult, the IVC may be represented below the level of the renal veins by two symmetrical vessels. The incidence is reported at 0.3% (Trigaux *et al.* 1998).

The azygos vein frequently arises from the posterior IVC at or below the level of the renal veins. A guidewire can pass into the azygos vein which then passes superiorly immediately in front of the spine before draining into the SVC, particularly in situations when the azygos vein is abnormally large. This can occur congenitally (with an incidence of 0.1%) or if the IVC is blocked (Trigaux *et al.* 1998) or in the presence of portal hypertension secondary to liver failure.

Rarely patients present with *dextrocardia*. In this condition, the heart's orientation is reversed so that it lies to the right of the midline. It is estimated to occur in 1 in 10 000 births. It can be associated with the reversal of abdominal/chest organs and blood vessels, so called situs inversus, in which case the SVC and IVC also lie to the left of the midline (Saha 2004) (Figure 2.5).

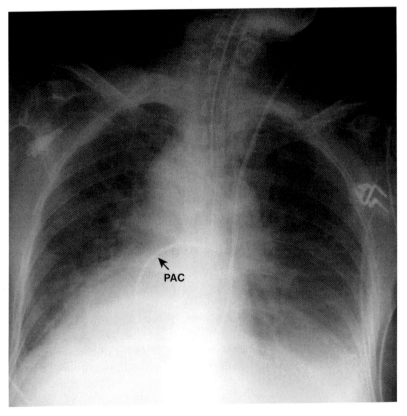

Figure 2.5 Dextrocardia with situs inversus. A pulmonary artery catheter (PAC) has been passed via the left internal jugular vein. It passes into the SVC and RA on the left and then into the RV (whose cavity it outlines, arrow) and to the pulmonary artery. A right subclavian catheter has also been inserted. Visceral inversion was seen by the presence of a nasogastric tube tracking to the right below the diaphragm. This was an incidental finding in an ICU patient with acute lung injury.

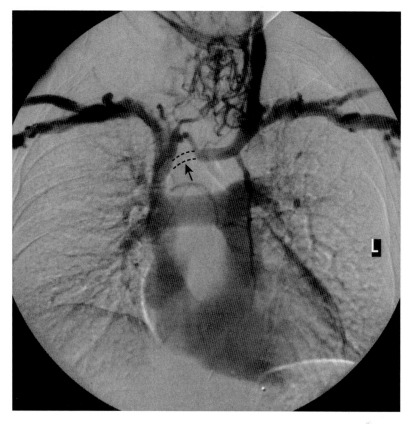

Figure 2.6 Intravenous contrast has been simultaneously injected into both arms. There is blockage of the left innominate vein (arrow) outlined by the dotted lines. Venous return from the left refluxes up the neck and returns to the SVC via numerous collaterals in the neck.

Acquired

Any patient with a history of previous central vein cannulation potentially has an acquired abnormality. Stenosis or thrombosis is common, particularly if the catheter remains in the patient for a prolonged time, or has been used for sclerosant solutions. For example, it has been estimated that a vascular stricture occurs in half the patients requiring subclavian venous access for haemodialysis (Hernandez 1998). This can present as failure to thread the guidewire or cannulae. Diagnosis of such problems can be confirmed by angiography or Doppler ultrasound studies (Figures 2.6 and 2.7). With advanced age and disease, the SVC and other great veins that may become increasingly tortuous (Figure 2.8) to cause difficulty with passage of guidewires and catheters.

Mediastinal shift from effusions, lung collapse or pneumonectomy will shift all structures including the SVC from the midline. This may cause confusion on X-rays if such abnormalities are not appreciated (Figure 2.9).

SVC compression from tumour is well recognised in oncology patients who develop signs of oedema and venous engorgement of the upper body. It is questionable whether a catheter should be passed through such a compressed vein as it may precipitate

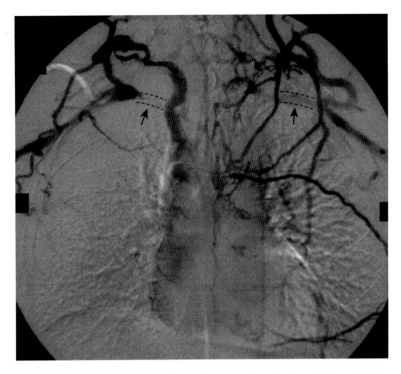

Figure 2.7 Intravenous contrast has been simultaneously injected into both arms. There is blockage of the right and left subclavian veins (arrows) following sclerosant chemotherapy. Contrast refluxes into the neck veins and passes centrally through numerous collaterals.

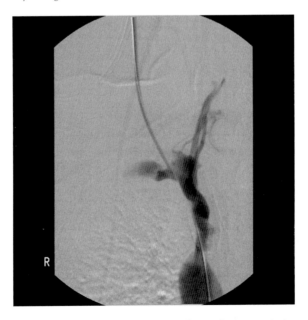

Figure 2.8 Great veins do not always run the straight course depicted in anatomical texts. This digital subtraction venogram in an elderly patient shows a tortuous SVC. It may be difficult to achieve passage of guidewires or good tip position in such cases.

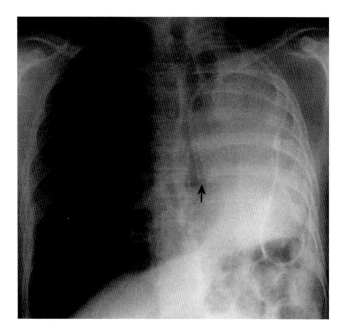

Figure 2.9 A Hickman catheter has been passed by the left subclavian route into the SVC. The catheter tip is marked with an arrow. The patient has gross mediastinal shift to the left following a previous left pneumonectomy, some years previously. The position of the catheter in the great veins may cause confusion unless the abnormal anatomy is appreciated.

total SVC obstruction. Furthermore, these patients are at particular risk of thrombosis and frequently cannot lie flat for procedures, due to dyspnoea. Short-term use of the femoral route (see Chapter 6) may be a safer option. Similar problems may also arise in the IVC.

Where should the catheter tip lie?

This has been the subject of recent debate (Fletcher and Bodenham 2000, Albrecht *et al.* 2004). However, some generalisations can be made regarding catheter tip position:

- The vein should be wide with a high blood flow so that drugs are diluted and therefore less likely to cause damage to the vein.
- The end of the catheter should be in the long axis of the vein rather than abutting the vessel wall, to minimise wall damage and inaccurate pressure readings. Vessel junctions should therefore be avoided.
- The catheter tip should be beyond the last venous valve in the route of access.

This narrows down the choice for long-term catheters. The tip can lie in the brachiocephalic veins, the upper or lower superior vena cava, the upper or lower inferior vena cava or the upper right atrium. The smaller the vein, the greater is the risk of wall damage.

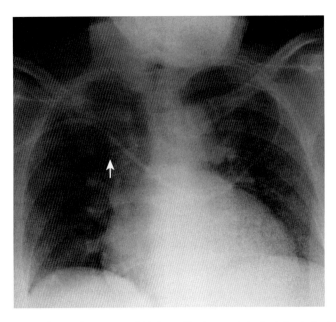

Figure 2.10 Chest X-ray of a poorly positioned Hickman line inserted via the left subclavian vein. The catheter blocked soon after insertion. The tip abuts the right wall of the SVC (arrow). This needs to be either withdrawn or advanced further into the SVC. In practice, it may be easier and safer to reposition from another site of access.

Safe positioning of catheters inserted from the left side of the chest may be particularly difficult. This is because there are more twists and turns to be negotiated as the brachiocephalic vein enters the SVC. Frequently, the catheter is left too short and the tip abuts the right wall of the SVC immediately as it enters the vein rather than passing down to lie in the long axis of the SVC/RA (Figure 2.10). This causes pain on infusion of irritant drugs and potentially serious vessel wall damage. It will also cause problems with aspiration of blood and interfere with accurate pressure monitoring from the distal port.

Debate exists as to whether the catheter tip should be allowed to lie inside the pericardium which extends from the heart to the lower SVC and upper IVC. Some argue that the tip should always be positioned outside the pericardium because if vessel wall perforation occurs, then bleeding or fluid infusion into the pericardium will produce cardiac tamponade. This can rapidly kill the patient. There have been repeated small numbers of such cases reported in the literature (Orme *et al.* 2007). An alternative view is that the advantages of a more central vein (such as a lesser risk of thrombosis) outweigh this relatively rare complication, and recommend placement in the lower SVC, upper right atrium or upper IVC. The pericardial reflection in relation to the SVC is very unlikely to extend above the carina (Albrecht *et al.* 2004). As long as the catheter tip is not inferior to the carina on an X-ray, it is unlikely to lie within the pericardium. A balanced view on positioning needs to be taken for each individual patient (Fletcher and Bodenham 2000) (see Table 2.1 and Figure 2.11). The pericardium does, however, ascend higher up the arch of the aorta and its branches, leading to the risk of tamponade if such arteries are inadvertently punctured during attempted venous cannulation.

Table 2.1 Catheter tip positions; refer to Figure 2.11 for description.

Catheter tip position	Zone in diagram	Advantages	Disadvantages
Left brachiocephalic	C	Outside pericardium Left-sided catheters tips can be pulled back to this position	Smaller vein Close to junctions Unsuitable for long-term use, sclerosant drugs or high-volume flows
Upper SVC	B	Outside pericardium Ideal for right-sided catheters	Tip of left-sided catheters can abut SVC vein wall end on
Upper right atrium	A	Larger vessel with optimum flows (dialysis catheters) Tip position suitable for all routes of access	Inside pericardium Arrhythmias or tricuspid valve damage can occur if catheter migrates inwards Risk of tamponade if perforation occurs

Reproduced with permission from *British Journal of Anaesthesia* (Stonelake and Bodenham 2006).

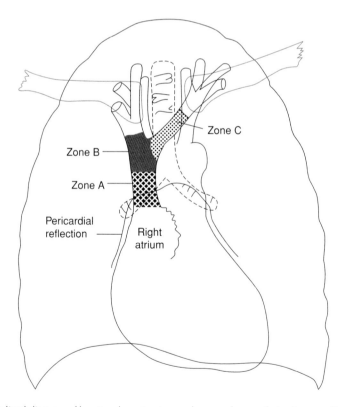

Figure 2.11 Stylised diagram of heart and great veins, and areas where catheter tips may lie (angles between veins may be more acute in vivo). (Reproduced with permission from *British Journal of Anaesthesia*, Stonelake and Bodenham 2006). See Table 2.1 for explanation.

Microanatomy

The first point to make about the microanatomy of veins is perhaps obvious – they are fragile structures. This fragility can have important consequences during the trauma of cannulation.

Wall thickness

Venous walls are thinner and more distensible than arteries due to the comparative weakness of the muscular middle coat. This allows the venous system to be very compliant and act as a blood reservoir. Veins have a wall thickness of roughly one-tenth or less compared to the internal diameter. For example, the wall thickness of a 5-mm-diameter vein is approximately 0.5 mm, whereas a similar sized artery would have a wall 1.5 mm thick. Veins inferior to the heart have thicker walls than those superior, presumably as a result of the greater hydrostatic pressure that they have to endure in the erect posture.

Components of vein walls

The walls of veins can be considered histologically in three sections: an inner endothelial layer, a middle muscular layer and an outer connective tissue layer. Classically, these are referred to as the tunica intima (endothelial), the tunica media (fibro-muscular) and the tunica adventitia (connective tissue) (Figure 2.12). Tunica is Latin for a cloak or tunic. The inner tunica intima layer is a delicate smooth layer of endothelial cells supported on a connective tissue bed which has a longitudinal organisation (Figure 2.13). The middle tunica media has a circumferential orientation of muscle fibres within elastic tissue. The outer tunica adventitia is a connective tissue coat, again with a longitudinal organisation.

Although all these layers are not distinct in all veins, an important functional point is that venous walls have a much larger proportion of outer connective tissue layer, and a smaller proportion of middle muscular tissue, compared to arterial walls. This makes them weaker as well as thinner than arteries. In addition, the longitudinal organisation of the main components of venous walls (the intima and adventitia layers) means that when veins are traumatised they have a tendency to tear along the long axis of the vein. Thus poor technique, particularly during dilatation of the vein, can cause large defects with serious bleeding consequences.

Adjacent structures

Veins tend to run with other structures in the body, particularly arteries, nerves and lymphatic vessels, which are therefore automatically at risk of inadvertent trauma when the vein is approached with a needle (see Chapter 12).

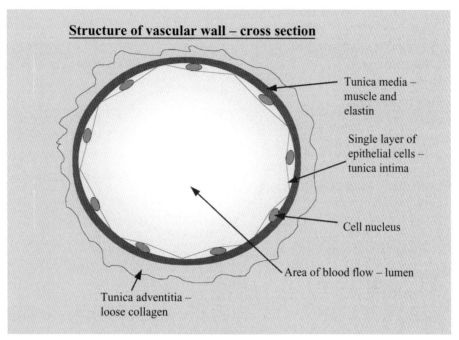

Figure 2.12 Stylised diagram of cross-section of vein wall.

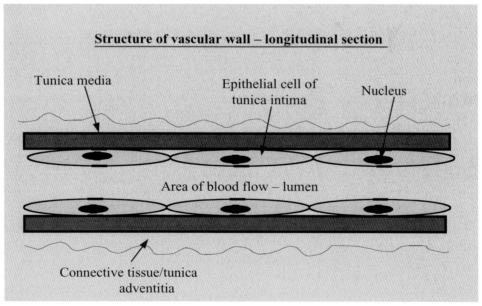

Figure 2.13 Longitudinal aspect of vein wall.

Choosing the best approach to the best vein

Choosing the best vein depends on many factors. These are influenced by both the patient characteristics and the purpose of the catheter to be inserted. The following major factors should be taken into account:

- Infection risk
- Thrombotic risk
- Risk of stenosis
- Bleeding risk
- Risk of pneumothorax
- Ease of tunnelling and port access
- Ease of insertion
- Clinical stability
- Experience and skill or operator
- Availability and expertise in the use of ultrasound screening and X-ray

Risk of infection (see also Chapter 13)

Infections are more common in the femoral region than in other common approaches. This is probably due to the proximity of the perineum and groin skin creases. Cannulation of the subclavian vein probably causes less infection than the internal jugular vein (McGee 2003). This is perhaps due to the proximity of the latter to the mouth or tracheostomy site in a critically ill patient. The presence of beards and movements of the neck make maintenance of a sterile dressing more challenging (Hall 2005). Infection at the skin entry site is an absolute contraindication for catheter insertion.

Risk of thrombosis and embolisation (see also Chapter 12)

Of the common approaches, the risk of thrombosis is lowest in the internal jugular vein, slightly higher in the subclavian vein and higher still in the femoral vein (Timsit *et al.* 1998, Merrer 2001, McGee 2003). Classically, thrombosis is more likely where there is the combination of low blood flow, turbulence and increased coagulopathy. It is therefore important to avoid small veins and junctions within the venous system. Having said this, the risk of embolus of any clot also varies with location. For example, thrombosis of superficial veins in the forearm causes mild morbidity, whereas femoral venous thrombosis may cause life-threatening pulmonary embolus. For this reason, femoral lines should be avoided wherever possible in patients at high risk of deep vein thrombosis.

Puncture of the carotid artery during attempted internal jugular vein cannulation can cause emboli of atherosclerotic tissue into the brain with the severe consequences of a stroke. The presence of a carotid bruit is a worry if not an absolute contraindication for this approach if performed without ultrasound guidance. The consequences of arterial emboli from the subclavian and femoral regions are likely to be much less severe to the patient.

Risk of vein stenosis

Stenosis of veins occurs after damage to the vein wall over a period of time. This can be due to infection, mechanical stress from the catheter itself (particularly a large device placed within a small vessel) or the infusion of solutions at a rate too high for the blood flow in the vein. It is particularly a consequence of long-term catheters and is potentially life limiting as vascular access becomes more and more difficult in these patients. The risks of stenosis reduce if the catheter lies in the centre of a big vein with a high blood flow away from junctions with other veins.

Risk of bleeding

Veins tend to run alongside arteries. This means that arterial puncture is a common risk during vein cannulation. The risk of arterial puncture is greater for the femoral vein than for the internal jugular vein, and less for the subclavian vein (McGee 2003, Hall 2005). However, this ranking is reversed when the consequences of arterial puncture are considered. The consequences of subclavian arterial puncture (or even tearing of the subclavian vein) can be considerable as the vessels cannot be compressed manually from the outside of the body because they lie under the clavicle and leads to haemothorax in severe cases. Bleeding into the neck following internal jugular vein cannulation attempts can cause life-threatening consequences such as airway obstruction, although at least these vessels can be compressed. In fact, the femoral vein is often the best approach in the patient with decreased blood clotting as a low approach below the inguinal ligament rarely causes life-threatening bleeding (Hall 2005). Cannulation of arms veins (basilic, cephalic and brachial) and passage into a central vein is a useful alternative in this setting.

Risk of pneumothorax (see also Chapter 12)

The risk of pneumothorax is greatest in the subclavian area due to the proximity of the pleura to the vein. Most studies report a rate of pneumothorax with this approach in the order of 2–3% (McGee 2003). The pleura can also be damaged during the anterior approach to the axillary vein as it lies a few centimetres beyond the vein in the direction needle movement. This approach is normally performed under real-time ultrasound guidance to reduce this risk. The only study to date using ultrasound guidance reported no pneumothoraces in 194 patients (Sharma 2004). Although less common, attempted cannulation of the internal jugular vein can also cause pleural breach as the pleural reflection can ascend as superiorly into the neck as a variation of normal anatomy.

Ease of subcutaneous tunnelling and access to ports

The subclavian area provides the easiest and shortest route for tunnelling to the chest wall. The jugular route is more uncomfortable during tunnelling over the clavicle, and more than one puncture site may be needed to facilitate tunnelling and avoid catheter kinking. A useful alternative is posterior tunnelling onto the shoulders with the device exiting onto the back which avoids these problems. It can make aseptic access to the injection ports difficult, particularly when self-administration is required. Femoral catheters can be tunnelled to the umbilical level on the abdomen.

Large breasts, breast implants, tumour recurrence, burns or other abnormalities may require innovative solutions as to where the catheter exits (see Chapters 3 and 11).

Ease of insertion and suitability for ultrasound guidance

Some veins are easier to access than others. The easiest veins to access are large, straight and either visible to the naked eye or consistently related to visible or palpable anatomical structures. As no veins constantly satisfy these criteria, ultrasound guidance is becoming increasingly popular. It has been shown to reduce insertion complications in some clinical trials and is currently recommended by The National Institute for Clinical Excellence (2002). Some veins such as the internal jugular are particularly suited to ultrasound scanning. Other veins cannot be seen at all as ultrasound cannot pass

Table 2.2 Common approaches.

Vein cannulated	Advantages	Disadvantages
Subclavian vein	Lower infection risk	Higher bleeding risk
	Suitability for subcutaneous tunnelling and port access	Higher pneumothorax risk
		'Blind' procedure that cannot be guided with ultrasound
Internal jugular vein	Vein can be seen clinically or with ultrasound	Medium infection risk
		Medium bleeding risk
	Convenient access during anaesthesia	Difficult to tunnel conveniently
	Right side highest probability of correct blind catheter tip placement	Difficult to dress
		Uncomfortable when not tunnelled
Femoral vein	Lower bleeding risk	Higher infection risk
	Patient can remain sitting during insertion	Higher thrombosis risk
		Poor catheter performance when patient sits up
Basilic vein	Lower bleeding risk	Medium thrombosis risk
	May be placed at bedside	Medium stenosis risk
	Patient can remain sitting during insertion	Basilic vein often thrombosed in long-term patients
	Probable lower infection risk	Passage into SVC occasionally difficult
	Ease of port access	Long catheter needed

through structures such as bone. The most important example of this is the subclavian vein which lies under the clavicle. An alternative in this region is the anterior approach to the axillary vein performed under ultrasound guidance.

The best approach

It can be seen that the choice of approach can be a complicated process. Advantages and disadvantages are summarised in Tables 2.2 and 2.3. In general, long-term tunnelled catheters are placed by the internal jugular, subclavian vein or axillary vein (anterior

Table 2.3 Less common approaches.

Vein cannulated	Advantages	Disadvantages	Insertion issues
Axillary vein (anterior approach)	Lower infection risk Lower thrombosis risk Low pneumothorax risk Suitability for tunnelling and port access	Medium bleeding risk	Ideally ultrasound guided through anterior chest wall
Axillary vein (lateral approach)	Superficial vessel for cannulation Useful for morbidly obese patients	Probable higher infection risk Uncomfortable when not tunnelled	Approached through the armpit Long catheter needed
External jugular vein	As for Internal Jugular vein Easy to cannulate	As for internal jugular vein	Can be difficult to pass through into subclavian and brachiocephalic veins
Brachial vein	As for Basilic vein	As for Basilic vein	Cannulated in mid upper arm with ultrasound guidance (Sandhu 2004) As for Basilic vein
Cephalic vein	As for Basilic vein	As for Basilic vein	Cephalic vein often thrombosed in long-term patients Passage into SVC frequently difficult Long catheter needed
Brachiocephalic (or supraclavicular approach to subclavian)	Easy access during anaesthesia Large target vein	As for subclavian vein	Supraclavicular approach

approach). For short- to medium-term access in hospital, the internal jugular and brachial veins are popular. For patients with coagulopathy or respiratory instability, the femoral vein and arms veins (basilic, cephalic or brachial) are useful. Complicated patients require a more creative approach.

Conclusions

The tip of most central catheters should lie in the central veins near the heart. The anatomy of these vessels is both variable and invisible to the naked eye. Therefore, a sound knowledge of the normal anatomy and common variants is an important aspect of competence for the clinician involved in the placement of such catheters.

The exact position of the catheter tip is controversial. Whether it should lie within or outside the pericardial reflection depends on the access route and the individual patient. What is not controversial is that it should lie in the long axis of a wide vein with a high blood flow, away from both the vessel wall and junctions.

The choice of access route depends on patient factors, the experience of the operator and the indication for the device. The aim is to achieve satisfactory function whilst minimising the risks which vary between both patients and approaches.

References

Albrecht K, Nave H, Breitmeier D et al. (2004). Applied anatomy of the superior vena cava. *British Journal of Anaesthesia* 92:75–77.

Fletcher SJ, Bodenham AR (2000). Safe placement of central venous catheters: where should the tip of the catheter lie? *British Journal of Anaesthesia* 85:188–191.

Ghadiali N, Teo LM, Sheah K (2006). Bedside confirmation of a persistent left superior vena cava based on aberrantly positioned central venous catheter on chest radiograph. *British Journal of Anaesthesia* 96:53–56.

Hall AP, Russell WC (2005). Toward safer central venous access: ultrasound guidance and sound advice. *Anaesthesia* 60:1–4.

Hernandez D, Diaz F, Rufino M et al. (1998). Subclavian vascular access stenosis in dialysis patients: natural history and risk factors. *Journal of the American Society of Nephrology* 9:1507–1510.

McGee DC, Gould MK (2003). Preventing complications of central venous catheterization. *New England Journal of Medicine* 85:584.

Merrer J, De Jonghe B, Golliot F et al. (2001). Complications of femoral and subclavian venous catheterization in critically ill patients. *Journal of American Medical Association* 286:700–707.

National Institute for Clinical Excellence (NICE) (2002). Guidance on the use of ultrasound locating devices for central venous catheters (NICE technology appraisal No. 49). London, UK.

Orme RM, McSwiney MM, Chamberlain-Webber RF et al. (2007). Fatal cardiac tamponade as a result of a peripherally inserted central venous catheter: a case report and review of the literature. *British Journal of Anaesthesia* 99:384–388.

Saha M, Chalil S, Sulke N (2004). Situs inversus and acute coronary syndrome. *Heart* 90:e20.

Sandhu NP, Sidhu DS (2004). Mid-arm approach to basilic and cephalic vein cannulation using ultrasound guidance. *British Journal of Anaesthesia* 93:292–294.

Sharma A, Bodenham AR, Mallick A (2004). Ultrasound guided infraclavicular axillary vein cannulation for central vein access. *British Journal of Anaesthesia* 93:188–192.

Stonelake P, Bodenham A (2006). The carina as a radiological landmark for central venous catheter tip position. *British Journal of Anaesthesia* 96:335–340.

Timsit JF, Farkas JC, Boyer JM *et al.* (1998). Central vein catheter related thrombosis in intensive care patients. *Chest* 114:207–213.

Trigaux JP, Vandroogenbroek S, De Wispelaere JF *et al.* (1998). Congenital anomalies of the inferior vena cava and left renal vein: evaluation with spiral CT. *Journal of Vascular and Interventional Radiology* 9:339–345.

Chapter 3

Patient examination and assessment: choice of devices

Helen Hamilton

Introduction

The insertion of a peripherally inserted vascular access device, performed by experienced healthcare professionals is considered routine and associated with few complications. However, for the less experienced the insertion of a central venous access device (CVAD) can be hazardous, resulting in occasionally severe or lethal consequences, many of which could be avoided if a correct clinical assessment is performed prior to the insertion of a CVAD.

The aim of this chapter is to encourage operators to consider issues that will aid in the safe insertion of a CVAD and limit the number of associated complications. The clinical order that such issues are addressed will vary from case to case. Patient assessment includes identifying not only the most suitable vein but also which intravenous medications the patient will require for their clinical needs and by which route these can be delivered. Factors to consider in relation to catheter selection include the proposed duration of therapy, whether therapies are vesicant, the volume of therapy to be infused and whether treatment will be delivered in hospital, or in the patient's home (Gabriel and Bravery 2005).

As more patients become recipients of a CVAD, particularly for intermediate to long-term parenteral therapies, it is important to ensure their clinical and social needs are met. Many patients may be clinically stable; however, others may be acutely unwell and therefore at greater risk of complications during the insertion of a device.

A number of routes have been described for cannulating central veins and for each of these routes a variety of techniques have been used and are described within this book. The wide choice of routes can often make the decision to determine the safest technique and most suitable route for the individual patient difficult. In practice, decisions are commonly taken on empirical grounds, but consideration of certain relevant factors can enable a more rational approach to be made.

Information and informed consent

Patient education is important because without patient cooperation complications and dissatisfaction are likely to occur. Patients should receive verbal and written information which is specific to the type of device and clinical situation. Patient information should include the following sections: (a) What is a CVAD? (b) What are the advantages and disadvantages of having a CVAD? (c) What are the risks involved in the insertion of a CVAD? (d) Care of the device and (e) Removal of the device.

Wherever possible, the patient should be involved in the decision-making process, to decide which device and vein would be most appropriate to meet their needs. Photographs or diagrams demonstrating the different types of devices and routes of access can be useful for patients to appreciate the options, although the clinical situation will usually dictate the best compromise. In the anaesthetised or critically ill patient issues of consent, patient information and cooperation are different, but a careful assessment of the patient is still necessary.

Informed consent is the act of obtaining a patient's permission to proceed with a procedure or treatment indicated for medical care, after an appropriate explanation of the treatment or procedure has been provided to the patient (Intravenous Nurses Society (INS) 2000, NICE 2003). This includes provision of information regarding the risks, the benefits, alternatives and the likely course of the patient's condition. The patient should be provided with written information on the CVAD insertion procedure, catheter management and potential complications. The patient's written consent for the procedure should either be gained on a form designed for that purpose or by verbal witnessed consent that is documented in the patient's records (DOH 2002).

All information must be provided in a manner consistent with the level of comprehension of the patient and in the language the patient or the health care surrogate is able to understand. Patients are often very knowledgeable regarding any long-term venous access, providing useful and relevant information to the operator regarding previous CVAD insertions and any complications or difficulties that may have occurred.

Allergies

Systemic and topical allergies appear to be becoming more common. The most frequently encountered allergy in relation to CVAD insertion is to different types of dressings as well as cleansing solutions latex and X-ray contrast. The patient must be asked about existing allergies and alternatives need to be found for any substance that is allergenic. True allergy to local anaesthetics is very rare, closer questioning will usually reveal bad experiences at the dentist or elsewhere with no hard evidence of anaphylaxis or other severe reactions. There are different classes of local anaesthetic drugs that can be used if the allergy appears significant. Applying a skin barrier prior to the dressing can reduce dressing allergies. In the case of latex allergies, as well as wearing latex-free gloves, the operator should be aware that some ultrasound probe covers also contain latex and an alternative must be found. Seek information as to the severity of the allergy as this varies from commonly encountered mild skin rashes to the very rare severe anaphylaxis. Should an allergy develop, appropriate medical advice should be sought, and alternative substances used.

Choice of anaesthetic techniques

Early assessment of patient anxiety and response to the suggestion of CVAD placement will aid the operator in deciding on the most appropriate anaesthetic technique. The types of anaesthesia and/or sedation that will be necessary and can be offered, for the insertion of that particular device should be explained. This varies and may involve only topical anaesthesia in the case of peripherally inserted central catheter (PICC) insertion or injection of subcutaneous local anaesthetic. Topical local anaesthetic creams are also useful for patient preparation prior to injection of local anaesthetic. The use of conscious sedation during CVAD insertion is commonplace and will vary according to local protocols, but should be set up in conjunction with the anaesthetic team to comply with the current guidelines (Royal College of Anaesthetists 2001). Conscious sedation is a state of minimally depressed level of consciousness, using single drugs such as midazolam, or a combination of drugs, which retain the patient's ability to maintain a patent airway independently and continuously, and respond appropriately to physical stimulation and verbal commands. It is important to remember that sedation alone does not reduce pain and therefore adequate local anaesthetic must be used in combination with sedative drugs. Occasional adults and most younger children will require a general anaesthetic for the insertion of a CVAD.

Physical examination and assessment

During the process of physical assessment much may be gained by initial observation when first meeting the patient. General physique, frame, height, weight, physical features such as bull neck, large breasts, goitres, stomas and open wounds may influence the final decision as to which access point the operator will use. Skeletal issues, e.g. kyphosis, should raise the operator's awareness in deciding upon the safest route and location for placement of a CVAD and one that may minimise the risk of secondary complications. For example, patients with a short thick neck (bull neck) may also present a challenge for the location of anatomical landmarks in the absence of ultrasound, when using the internal jugular route (Figure 3.1). Complications caused by relevant anatomical issues may include perforation of the proximal superior vena cava (SVC) caused by advancing the introducer of a CVAD too medially into the subclavian vein in a small patient.

In addition to clinical issues, consideration should also be given to the cosmetic outcome of catheter placement in the case of longer-term access. Discussion with the patient in terms of clothing preferences, e.g. dress/shirt necklines, work and leisure activities can guide the operator to the most suitable and most cosmetically acceptable position for the patient. Care should be taken to avoid the catheter exiting near the axilla, due to increased risk of infection, or exposed areas such as the 'V' shaped anterior chest wall and cleavage of a female.

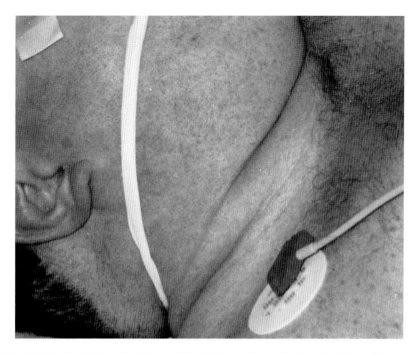

Figure 3.1 A bull neck with loss of surface markings in the neck. Landmark-guided internal jugular puncture is more difficult in such cases.

Vascular assessment

The operator should perform a physical assessment of the anatomical areas for proposed cannulation and note any history of previous central venous catheterisation. If there has been evidence of a venous thrombosis caused by the presence of a CVAD, it may be prudent to perform ultrasound (with or without Doppler) of the affected site to exclude thrombus and ensure vein patency.

Knowledge of normal anatomy of peripheral and central veins and their variants is essential. A history and clinical signs of thrombosis, venous stenosis and anatomical anomalies are all relevant, and prior knowledge may avoid unsuccessful catheter placement and long-term complications. Any swelling of the upper and lower limbs or head and neck should raise the suspicion of a deep vein thrombosis. Lymphoedema is another common cause for swollen limbs.

Visual examination of the thorax, abdomen, upper and lower limbs, and neck may reveal the presence of dilated collateral veins and swelling, suggesting the presence of thrombosis or stenosis of major underlying veins (Figure 3.2). Such venous collaterals develop and enlarge over time to provide an alternative route for venous drainage back to the heart (see further images in Chapters 2, 10 and 11), and can on occasions provide a route of access in the more challenging case. Such collaterals are readily seen in deeper tissues with ultrasound. Further radiological investigations may be required to provide evidence of the cause of these clinical presentations.

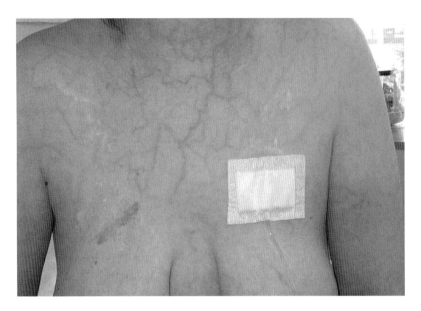

Figure 3.2 Dilated collateral veins over the chest wall and breast in a patient with an underlying blocked SVC following long-term venous access. Note scars from multiple previous access procedures. The presence of such veins should warn the operator of the presence of blocked central veins.

A history of deep vein thrombosis, pulmonary embolism or inferior vena cava filter insertion greatly increases the risk of subsequent catheter-related thrombosis in the longer term. Consideration should be given as to the optimal site of access to reduce this risk (usually the right internal jugular), choice of catheter, optimum catheter tip position and the need for therapeutic dose anticoagulation whilst the catheter is in situ.

Cool or discoloured extremities with a poor peripheral circulation may result from peripheral arterial disease. Scars may reveal previous arterial surgery with vein or prosthetic graft material in situ (e.g. carotid endarterectomy or femoral bypass). In general, such sites should be avoided for venous access as any arterial damage, other procedural complication or local sepsis would be likely to have devastating consequences on the arterial graft.

Assessment of respiratory function

Assessment of respiratory function will provide information that may influence the technique, site and the device used (Hamilton 1998). Breathless patients may be unable to tolerate laying flat or head down (Trendelenburg) position during insertion. For this group of patients, a PICC or simple peripheral venous access may be more suitable. A pneumothorax or other respiratory complication would be very poorly tolerated in such patients. A chest X-ray or CT of the chest, if indicated, prior to insertion of a CVAD may provide valuable information to guide the most appropriate site for insertion. Ventilated patients or those with emphysema/COPD may be at greater risk of pneumothorax during the insertion of a CVAD as a result of the hyperinflation of

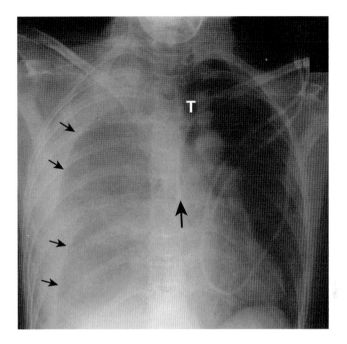

Figure 3.3 This patient has gross mediastinal shift secondary to a large malignant right pleural effusion (arrows mark lung edge). Such shift may cause difficulty in assessing catheter tip position for the inexperienced operator. A Hickman catheter has been inserted via the left axillary subclavian route to correctly lie in the SVC or upper right atrium which is just to the left of the midline due to mediastinal shift (tip thick arrow). T, tracheal air shadow.

the lungs. The subclavian route may be more risky in such patients unless ultrasound guidance is used. A pneumothorax is much more likely to tension in the presence of positive pressure ventilation. If a pneumothorax is already present, then consider using this side for central venous access rather than the other undamaged side which already has the pneumothorax present.

Patients with longstanding respiratory disease may have considerable distortion of mediastinal structures with shift of the SVC making assessment of tip position difficult, e.g. larger effusions, pulmonary collapse or post pneumonectomy (Figure 3.3).

Cardiovascular

Increasing numbers of patients have implanted pacemakers and defibrillators, usually inserted via the subclavian veins and SVC into the right heart. These do not represent absolute contraindications to central venous catheters (CVCs), but a careful assessment of risk benefits should be taken. There is a small but finite risk of catheters interfering with the position of leads of these devices and infection of such devices from CVCs would lead to major problems. The access site should be on the opposite side to where the implanted box lies wherever possible (Figure 3.4). Patients may have difficulty in lying flat.

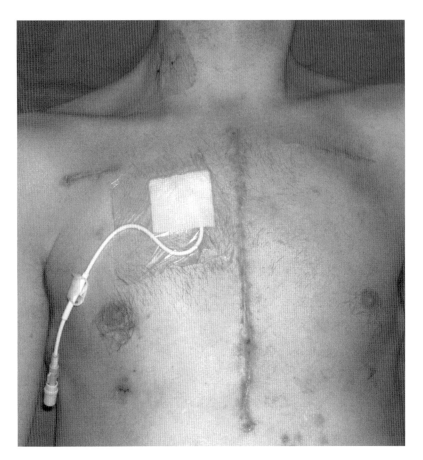

Figure 3.4 This patient has had recent surgery with a median sternotomy to replace his aortic root and an infected aortic valve. He remained fully anticoagulated with warfarin and an INR of 2.5. He has two recent scars from pacemaker boxes below each clavicle. A Hickman catheter has been inserted via the right internal jugular vein, with ultrasound guidance, and tunnelled between the scars on the chest wall.

Neurological

Patients with a depressed level of consciousness are at risk during interventional procedures. They may not lie still even with adequate local anaesthesia, and may be very sensitive to the effects of sedative or analgesic drugs. They may not tolerate head down positioning. Careful considerations of risk benefits should be taken and a proportion of cases may be better performed under general anaesthesia. In a paralysed limb, discomfort may not be felt by patient – leading to increased risk of unrecognised extravasation of drugs.

Fractures and arthritis

It is unwise to attempt a landmark-based subclavian approach in a patient with a previous fracture of the clavicle on the affected side, as it can be notoriously difficult, due to the calcification around the fracture. The CVAD is best placed on the opposite side to the fracture, or a jugular approach should be used. Recent fractures of the upper limb bones are a contraindication for PICC placement on the affected side.

Arthritis, particularly in the elbow, shoulder and neck joints, will make PICC insertion more challenging, as positioning the patient may cause pain and discomfort, making access of the great vessels technically very difficult. Advancement of the catheter around an arthritic shoulder is often unachievable. The use of ultrasound (NICE 2002) in the placement of PICCs has revolutionised practice for this group of patients and can be used to check if the catheter has migrated into other vessels, usually the internal jugular vein.

Fractures or congenital skeletal disorders involving the ribs, neck and spine are highly relevant to the operator when the insertion of a CVAD is being considered. Congenital deformities of the spine may distort the ideal patient position for CVAD insertion, which can at times be improved with the use of pillows etc. However, positioning a patient in an ideal position for the operator may not always be acceptable to the patient. If a compromise cannot be made, thought should be given to the safest approach if serious risks are to be avoided. This may require radiology or a surgical colleague's assistance.

Convex or concave sternums

A chest with a distorted sternum will greatly increase the risk of pneumothorax if the subclavian approach is attempted. The safest approach is to use the internal jugular vein.

Obesity

Excessive weight can also present the operator with technical difficulties. Placing the patient in the Trendelenburg position may result in some degree of respiratory compromise due to pressure on the diaphragm by a large abdomen. If this is a predicted outcome, then the patient should be left in a semi-recumbent position until it is absolutely necessary for the patient to adopt the Trendelenburg position, prior to cannulation.

The subclavian approach may be hampered due to reduced ability to locate the clavicles and to successfully cannulate the vein. Placing a rolled hand towel between the scapulae may facilitate the process. The jugular veins are usually full due to high venous pressure in such patients and are easily visualised with ultrasound in the semi-recumbent position, even in the most morbidly obese (Figure 3.5). The femoral veins are ideally avoided in such patients due the increased risk of thrombosis and DVT, and the marked intertrigo and candida infections which are commonly present.

Cachexia

Massive weight loss can also present the operator with challenges. The risk of a pneumothorax is increased when performing the subclavian approach, due to loss of subcutaneous tissue between the ribs and clavicle. The internal jugular approach may also be difficult, as the veins will be more mobile due to loss of subcutaneous tissue, and are very superficial. Make a small skin incision before inserting the needle to avoid passing

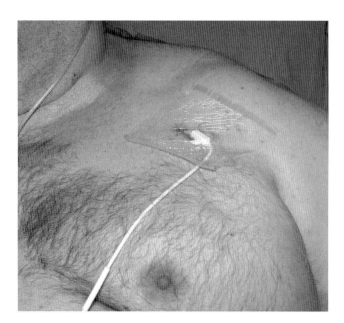

Figure 3.5 A Hickman line has been inserted via the left internal jugular in this morbidly obese man (BMI 55) for TPN following a leak after gastric stapling. He could not lie flat due to dyspnoea from pneumonia and his size, so the procedure was performed under local anaesthesia, in the sitting position. Surface landmarks were difficult to identify, and the carotid artery was difficult to palpate. The neck veins were well filled, even in the upright position, and easily visualised and cannulated under ultrasound guidance.

straight through the vein after pushing it through the skin. Tunnelling of the catheter may also present a challenge due to loss of subcutaneous tissue. Cuffs and catheters can erode out of the skin in such patients.

Large breasts

When the patient is placed in the Trendelenburg position, gravity will cause large breasts to obliterate any visible contour of the clavicle. Assistance will need to be sought to gently retract the breast tissue down, to enable the operator to better visualise landmarks and palpate the clavicle. Such assistance will also aid tunnelling of the catheter in both the subclavian and the internal jugular approaches. Care must be taken not to tunnel too deeply, as this will hinder removal of the device by the inability to palpate the cuff under deep subcutaneous tissue. When measuring the catheter length for tip position, it is advisable to allow extra length for displacement when the patient stands erect. The assistant should adopt maximum barrier precautions to ensure maximum sterility to the field.

Lymphoedema

Patients, who have had axillary lymph node resections, usually in association with breast surgery, are at high risk of developing lymphoedema of the affected arm, due to the reduction in lymph flow. Not even peripheral cannulation should be attempted in an affected limb due to the high risk of infection with even apparently trivial injury. The axillary/subclavian route on the affected side is ideally best avoided to reduce the risk of thrombosis in an already compromised limb. Similar considerations would apply to lymphoedema in the lower limbs.

Stomas, open wounds, tracheostomy

The presence of any of the above can present a potential risk of CVAD contamination. If possible, the insertion site should be on the opposite side to any potential source of contamination, and every effort made to tunnel the catheter away from the site. An example of this would include tunnelling a subclavian catheter across or behind the shoulder (Figures 3.6a and 3.6b). The proximal end of the catheter should be secured so that it does not touch the area to be avoided, and the bung should also be wrapped in sterile gauze to further prevent any contamination.

Bull neck

This term is applied to patients who have short, wide necks (Figure 3.1). This anatomy hinders internal jugular placement as anatomical landmarks are difficult to identify and ultrasound use may be awkward. Arterial puncture and puncture of the apical pleura is more likely. Tunnelling of the catheter will be difficult, due to the acute angle between the neck and chest wall. A subclavian approach may be preferable in this situation.

Skin and subcutaneous tissues

Previous surgical scars, previous access sites, burns, tumours, sites of infection and other skin disorders will all impact on the choice of vein access site and where any tunnelling and exit site should lie. Prosthetic breast implants are increasingly prevalent, and if catheters are tunnelled too close, they may be at risk of infection if catheter-related sepsis occurs.

Infection issues

Elevation of inflammatory markers or positive cultures from blood or other tissues should raise the question of whether a long-term or short-term device should be placed initially. An elevated temperature, white blood cell count or C-reactive protein suggest infection, and should influence the type and timing of CVAD insertion. A history of recent catheter-related sepsis at an individual site should prompt clinicians to avoid this site, if possible, until all signs of inflammation externally have cleared. Bear in mind that infected clot may remain invisible within the central veins for some time after the catheter has been removed. Advice from microbiology can be helpful in this situation, in assessing the relative risk of catheter-related sepsis or simpler colonisation, the timing of previous catheter removal, and antibiotic therapy prior to insertion. Temporary venous access may be preferable until the source of infection is located and treated effectively.

The optimum site for access will depend on the factors listed above and the physical state of the patient. An unconscious ventilated patient will frequently dribble potentially infected oropharyngeal or respiratory secretions onto the neck, making this site

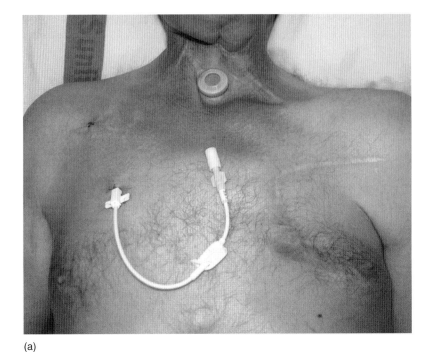

(a)

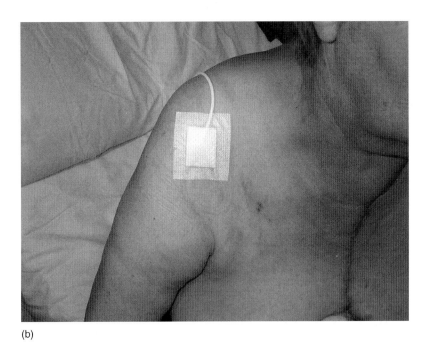

(b)

Figure 3.6 (a) Patient with permanent tracheostomy, radical neck dissection and free-flap reconstruction following laryngectomy for tumour. The right axillary subclavian approach was the only realistic site for insertion of a Hickman line that has been tunnelled away from the stoma. (Reproduced with permission from *Anaesthesia*, Galloway *et al.* 2005.) (b) Reverse subcutaneous tunnel over the shoulder to avoid CVAD contamination of a recent surgical site on the anterior chest wall.

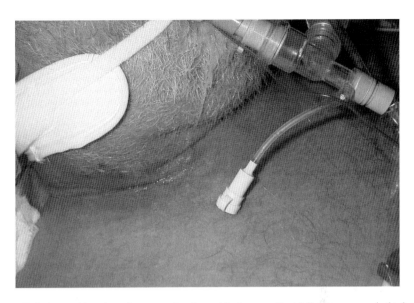

Figure 3.7 Right internal jugular vein access sites in a critical care patient following removal of infected catheters. Note the skin induration and soiling of the area by oropharyngeal secretions and ventilation and suction tubes.

potentially unattractive in this respect (Figure 3.7). Similar considerations apply to stomas (see above).

Where possible, the procedure should be performed in a clean clinical environment designated for CVAD insertion, e.g. an X-ray department, operating theatre or other procedure suite where a high standard of asepsis is practiced. Whatever the environment, maximal sterile barrier conditions (mask, cap, sterile gloves, gown and large drape) have been shown to lower the risk of acquiring catheter-related infections (Mermel *et al.* 1991, Raad *et al.* 1994) (Figure 3.8). Changing gloves immediately prior to catheter insertion is recommended and powder-free gloves are preferred (Elliott *et al.* 1994, RCN 2005). Published evidence shows, however, that the risk of infection depends mainly on the presence of bacteria on the skin (Fletcher and Bodenham 1999), hence skin cleansing is the most important part of care before CVAD insertion and allowing the skin to dry completely. Hair removal may be necessary prior to catheter insertion but close shaving should be avoided because of the potential for causing micro-abrasions which increase the risk of infection (RCN 2005); therefore, the use of clippers or scissors are preferred.

Radiological assessment

Most hospitalised patients have a large number of radiology images which may give useful information about anatomical abnormalities even if this was not the reason for the request for imaging. Review chest X-rays, ultrasound or CT images, plus their reports, of areas of anatomical interest, as it will not be defensible practice if you have a complication which could have been anticipated from already available imaging.

If there has been evidence of a venous thrombosis caused by the presence of a CVAD, it may be prudent to perform ultrasound (with or without Doppler) of the affected

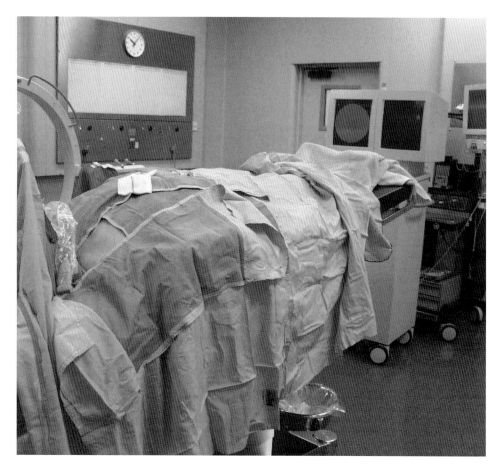

Figure 3.8 Patient prepared for vascular access procedure via right subclavian site in a theatre. Note head down tilt, wide drapes for asepsis, a bar lifts drapes to prevent claustrophobia, an ultrasound probe covered with a sterile sleeve.

site to exclude thrombus and ensure vein patency. This is increasingly performed by operators with bedside machines rather than formal radiology referrals.

Formal radiological assessment of the great vessels of the thorax/abdomen may be required prior to CVAD insertion, particularly if there is a history of difficult procedures in the past or clinical evidence suggests abnormalities may be present. These may include mediastinal shift (Figure 3.9), pacemakers, venous stenosis or tumours invading the central venous system (see radiology and Chapters 10 and 11).

Laboratory assessments

Biochemical assessment

Recent serum electrolytes should be within the normal range prior to insertion of a CVAD, in particular potassium, which if low or high may increase the risk of arrhythmias.

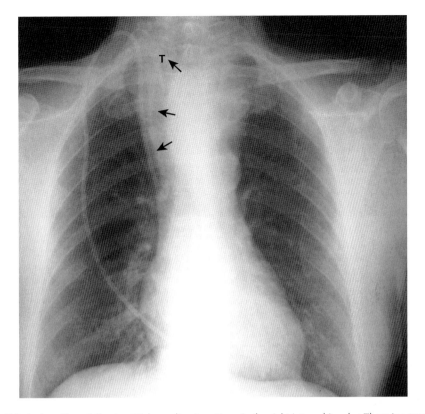

Figure 3.9 A chest X-ray following Hickman line insertion via the right internal jugular. There is a tumour in the upper mediastinum pushing (arrows) the trachea (black air shadow T) and catheter in the great veins over to the right.

Coagulation assessment

The risk of haemorrhage caused by accidental arterial puncture, a venous tear or from tunnel sites can be reduced by ensuring the patient has adequate coagulation status prior to commencing the procedure. For a scheduled insertion of a CVAD using the jugular, femoral or subclavian approach, the patient's coagulation status and platelet count should be checked against the normal range.

Normal values:
APTT: 22.0–34.0 s
PT: 10.5–13.5 s
Platelets: 150–400 $\times$ 10^9/l

Patients with a very low platelet count will require a platelet transfusion immediately prior to CVAD insertion to elevate their count to $>$70 $\times$ 10^9/l (BCSH 2003).

Those patients whose coagulation is deranged due to liver dysfunction or critical illness will require prothrombin concentrate, fresh frozen plasma, cryoprecipitate or other preparations; seek haematology advice.

Patients receiving warfarin therapy will need it to be either stopped or converted to heparin about 3 days beforehand – and their INR should be checked prior to catheter insertion. Typically, an INR of 1.5 or below should be achieved. The INR can be corrected more quickly with the use of vitamin K, prothrombin concentrate or fresh frozen plasma (BCSH 1990).

Intravenous unfractionated heparin is usually stopped 3 hours before insertion and restarted when haemostasis is secured. Low molecular weight heparins will require 12–24 hours after the last dose for the effects of therapeutic doses to clear. Prophylactic doses of low molecular weight heparin are usually continued.

Full correction of blood parameters may be undesirable and impossible to achieve in emergency situations or in some disease states. The risks and benefits of insertion of different types of CVCs at each site must be reviewed on an individual basis in these situations (see Figure 3.4). It will also depend on operator experience and local facilities. PICC placement may be safe in the presence of coagulation abnormalities because of the relative ease with which vessels in the arm can be compressed. Where the risk of bleeding is high, or where difficulties may be anticipated, experienced personnel and the use of ultrasound are strongly recommended (Hatfield and Bodenham 1999), because this increases the likelihood of an atraumatic, first pass procedure.

Patient factors which impact on the site of access are summarised in Table 3.1.

Catheter selection

Decision trees, algorithms and other types of flow charts can be instituted to aid in the intravenous catheter selection process. Ideally, the most appropriate catheter is placed early in the patient's treatment process allowing one device to be used for the entire length of therapy.

Information to determine the best catheter to use for each patient situation is available through the Center for Disease Control (CDC 2002), the NICE Guidelines (2003), Royal College of Nursing (RCN) Standards of Practice (RCN 2005) and Infusion Nurses Society (INS 2006). Each case is different and catheter selection may not be straightforward. Factors to consider are shown in Box 3.1.

Choice of CVAD

CVADs can be divided into (a) non-tunnelled catheters, (b) skin-tunnelled catheters, (c) implanted ports, (d) apheresis/dialysis catheters (tunnelled and non-tunnelled) and (e) PICCs. A representative sample of devices is discussed and illustrated in Chapter 4. They may have single or multiple lumens. Multiple-lumen catheters are advantageous in patients who are critically ill, or undergoing stem cell transplantation or chemotherapy where a number of drugs, fluids and blood products require simultaneous infusion. Multiple-lumen catheters are associated with increased morbidity (Farkas *et al.* 1992, Henriques *et al.* 1993, Dezfulian *et al.* 2003), but in many clinical situations, the increased risk is likely to be offset by the convenience of their use. If parenteral nutrition (PN) is being administered, use of a single-lumen catheter or lumen exclusively for that purpose is recommended (Pratt *et al.* 2001). In addition, it has been shown that smaller diameter catheters minimise the risk of catheter-related thrombosis and subsequent venous stenosis (Knutsad *et al.* 2003), and they are also less traumatic on insertion.

Table 3.1 Clinical assessment issues associated with CVC insertion.

Technical problem	Issue	Suggestion
Respiratory		
Tracheostomy ET tube IPPV	Cross infection from sputum onto CVAD	Reverse tunnel if tunnelled away from tracheostomy stoma
		Careful dressing technique and aseptic management of CVAD
COPD	Hyperinflated lungs	Consider high internal jugular approach.
	Consider high risk factors, e.g. pneumothorax.	Low threshold for drains if pneumothorax occurs. Use ultrasound
Intolerance of lying flat, due to pleural effusion, pulmonary oedema. Patient may be unable to lie in ideal position	Respiratory distress	Keep upright until immediately before cannulation. Utilise ultrasound.
Chest drain in situ		Utilise same side for IV access – minimise risk of damage to opposite lung. Seek most experienced operator
Skeletal system		
Kyphosis		
Arthritis of shoulders and neck	Avoid subclavian approach	Position patient with pillows to establish 'square' shoulder position and ensure comfort
Fracture clavicle	Patient may be unable to lie in ideal position	
	Bony calcification may reduce possibility of gaining venous access	Consider PICC
		Ultrasound
Gastrointestinal system		
Intestinal failure	Potential for long-term parenteral nutrition – high-risk stenosis or thrombosis if large diameter device used	Consider smallest bore device and discuss final position of device with patient, particularly if patient is planning to manage device
Stomas	Infection risk	Consider insertion of PICC under ultrasound guidance, gaining venous access as far distal as possible
		Ensure exit site of CVAD is diverted away from stoma
Neurological system		
Confusion	Consider displacement of device by patient	Reverse tunnel
		Secure suturing and dressing

(Continued)

Table 3.1 (*Continued*)

Technical problem	Issue	Suggestion
Hemiparesis	**Never** cannulate affected limb	Discomfort cannot be felt by patient – unrecognised extravasation a possibility
Epilepsy	Consider displacement and potential damage to CVAD	Consider reverse tunnel or PICC
Cardiovascular system (see text) Clarify current cardiac rhythm	Arrhythmia Low CVP – under filled may make gaining venous access difficult	Ventricular ectopics may occur if CVAD inserted into right atrium Avoid the subclavian on side housing the pacing box and wire
Consider patient's fluid status, e.g. low CVP	Volume resuscitate first, time with respiration with ultrasound, Valsalva or steep head down tilt	May require additional fluid if risk of air embolus is to be minimised
High CVP/heart failure **Renal system** Consider potential for creation of shunt/fistula at later stage	Patient cannot lie flat Renal patients potentially will require central venous access for life	Perform procedure semi-recumbent with ultrasound guidance PICC insertion should be avoided and only be considered after discussion with medical team responsible for patient Always use smallest device possible to reduce risk of stenosis and thus thrombosis (Sansivero 1998). Avoid subclavian as patent vein needed for fistula
Infection Assess source and site of infection	Insertion of long-term CVAD may encourage 'seeding' of organism onto CVAD	Consider either PICC or temporary non-tunnelled CVAD until symptoms of sepsis are under control.

This may require in some adults the use of devices originally designed for children, e.g. Broviac as opposed to Hickman lines.

Non-tunnelled catheters

Such devices are used in large numbers for acutely ill patients requiring fluid therapy and central venous pressure monitoring, major surgery and anaesthesia and other short-term uses in hospitalised patients.

In an attempt to reduce infection rates, various materials have been investigated. These have been reviewed in the Chapter 13, and antimicrobial/antiseptic impregnated catheters have been shown to be effective in reducing catheter colonisation and related

---

Box 3.1 Factors to consider in selection of the type of vascular access device.

- Type of medication to be used
- Osmolarity and pH of the solution to be infused
- Duration of therapy, intermittent or continuous
- Diagnosis of the patient
- Secondary risk factors, chronic diseases or problems that may affect the incidence of complications
- Patient preference, activities, job and lifestyle
- Financial resources to cover required therapies
- Future intravenous needs and long-term prognosis
- Current availability and status of peripheral veins
- History of neurological impairment
- Surgery affecting the veins or lymphatic system
- Coagulation problems
- Thrombosis history
- Previous catheter-threading problems

---

blood stream infections in a number of studies. More recent studies have been less convincing and the whole area is still contentious.

Skin-tunnelled catheters

Skin-tunnelled catheters are recommended for patients in whom long-term (>30 days) central venous access is anticipated (Pratt *et al.* 2001). They have been shown to have lower infection rates than those of non-tunnelled catheters (Randolph *et al.* 1998), because the combination of tunnelling and the presence of a Dacron cuff are thought to reduce infection. The cuff induces an inflammatory reaction leading to fibrosis with catheter fixation usually occurring within 3–4 weeks of insertion, and reduces the potential for skin organisms to advance up the subcutaneous tunnel and enter the vascular system. Silver impregnated Hickman-type catheters are now commercially available and undergoing clinical trials.

Subcutaneous ports

Ports have been shown to have the lowest reported rates of catheter-related blood stream infections compared to either tunnelled or non-tunnelled CVCs (Pegues *et al.* 1992, Groeger *et al.* 1993). Most ports are single lumen and the requirement for needle access makes them more suited to long-term intermittent therapy. They tend to be used more frequently in paediatrics and patients with solid tumours and those requiring long-term antibiotics (e.g. patients with cystic fibrosis) (Camp Sorrell 1992, Gabriel 1999). Port membranes deteriorate as a result of repeated punctures with a potential lifespan of 1000–2000 punctures depending on the needle gauge used to access the port. It is recommended the smallest non-coring needle be used as appropriate and changed every 7 days (RCN 2005). The principles of skin asepsis, insertion and accessing and flushing the hub also apply to fully implanted ports. If patients are accessing their own

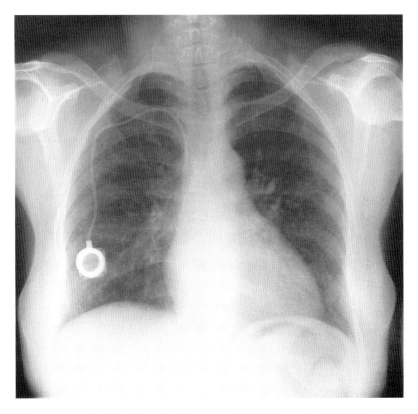

Figure 3.10 A post-procedure chest X-ray showing a port relatively low on the right chest wall inserted via the right axillary subclavian vein.

port then ideally it should be located low on the rib cage (Figure 3.10) or upper arm for easy access. When patients are not accessing their own device then the port is usually located on the upper rib cage near the clavicle. Ports near the sternum provide better needle stability and ease of access. Adequate subcutaneous tissue will prevent erosion through the skin. If the port is placed too deeply or there is excess adipose tissue, it can make access difficult. Placement under the arm, in the breast or the soft tissue of the abdomen should be avoided (Goodman 2000).

Dialysis/apheresis catheters

These can be either non-tunnelled or tunnelled, and a variety of types are commercially available for longer-term use. These are larger bore catheters and usually require the lumen volume to be filled with stronger solutions of heparin (e.g. heparin 1000 u/mL) to maintain patency. The volume instilled should equal the internal volume of each lumen (usually stated on device) to avoid systemic heparinisation of the patient. It should be noted that for optimal performance of this type of catheter, it is usually necessary to position the tip within the upper right atrium to achieve adequate flow rates (Veseley 2003).

Table 3.2 Types of commercially available catheters.

Catheter type	Advantages	Disadvantages	Typical uses	Dwell time
Non-tunnelled catheters	Easy to insert and remove Multiple lumens available	Short-term use Higher risk of infection	Fluid therapy Measurement CVP Antibiotics Vasoactive drugs	5–10 days depending on whether antimicrobial coating present
Skin-tunnelled catheters	Lower infection rates than non-tunnelled Long-term use	Surgical insertion and removal Expensive	Cancer chemotherapy Parenteral nutrition Blood products	6 weeks to years
Ports	Cosmetic benefit when in situ Patient can swim/bathe as normal Low maintenance Long-term use Lower infection rates than skin-tunnelled catheters	Surgical insertion and removal Expensive Larger scars Less suitable for frequent continuous access	Long-term antibiotics Access in children	3 months–years
Dialysis/apheresis catheters ● Non-tunnelled (e.g. Vascath^{TM}) ● Skin-tunnelled (e.g. Permcath^{TM}, Tesio^{TM})	Permits high blood flow rates for extracorporeal circuits Easy to insert and remove Lower infection rates than non-tunnelled Long-term use	Large bore Requires flushing with strong heparin (e.g. 1000 u/mL) Short-term use Surgical insertion and removal	Dialysis Apheresis Rapid volume transfusions	10–20 days to months/years
PICCs	Easy to insert and remove on general ward Do not require platelet support or correction of clotting prior to insertion/removal	Higher thrombosis rate particularly in polyurethane variety Slower flow rates particularly in silicone/valved varieties Catheter longevity is lower than skin-tunnelled devices Incidence of malposition is greater than in other types of CVC	Medium-term access for drugs, fluids, cancer chemotherapy	Have been known to last for a year

They are typically inserted via the right internal jugular vein to allow straight access to the SVC.

Peripherally inserted central catheters

PICCs represent a device type that can be considered to have an intermediary role in central venous access. These catheters are usually inserted at the bedside via a proximal basilic, cephalic or median antecubital vein and are available as single or multilumen catheters (see Chapter 8). They are well suited for ambulatory or outpatient therapy (Whitman 1996), short-term use in anaesthesia and surgery, rather than intensive inpatient therapy (Maki *et al.* 2005), and have been shown to have a higher incidence of thrombosis in patients with haematological malignancies (Cortelezzi *et al.* 2003). This is an important consideration in patients who have had previous thrombosis or if they are receiving medication, which may increase thrombophilic tendency, for example thalidomide therapy. PICCs can be made of either silicone rubber or polyurethane, the former being associated with a lower risk of thrombosis (Galloway and Bodenham 2004). PICCs are the first choice for central access whenever possible. The low cost of insertion and the low risk to the patient all point to the PICC line as an excellent option if a treatment plan exceeds 5 days, unstable clinical status prevails or if unable to maintain a short peripheral intravenous device.

The available types of catheter are summarised in Table 3.2. The decision as to which device is most suitable is based on diagnosis and length and type of therapy, patient preference, clinical status, availability of patent veins, operator experience and previous central venous access history (Hamilton & Fermo 1998, Hamilton 2000, Chernecky *et al.* 2002). Key principle is to avoid multiple catheterisations and to preserve vein patency.

Intravenous therapy requirements

The duration of therapy often impacts on the type of device selected. For example, a PICC is often suitable for a 4–6 week course of treatment, while a skin-tunnelled catheter would be more suitable for therapy required for 3–6 months or longer (Cole 1999) or an implanted port more appropriate for long-term intermittent intravenous access. Multiple therapies that are incompatible would not be appropriate for a single-lumen device. Equally, very viscous solutions often require a larger diameter device, which may exclude some PICCs.

Conclusion

An informed, thorough and expert assessment of individual patient requirements for central venous cannulation has the potential to significantly reduce the incidence of complications, improve the success rate of procedures and lead to increased patient satisfaction. These advantages extend beyond immediate insertion complications to easier management by hospital nursing and medical personnel, more appropriate selection, and ultimately the increased likelihood of successful management and treatment by the patient or carer in the community environment.

References

BCSH (1990). Guidelines on oral anticoagulation. *Journal of Clinical Pathology* 43:177–183.

BCSH (2003). Guidelines for the use of platelet transfusions. *British Journal of Haematology* 122:10–23.

Camp Sorrell D (1992). Implantable ports: everything you always wanted to know. *Journal of Intravenous Nursing* 15:262–273.

Center for Disease Control (2002). Guidelines for the prevention of intravascular catheter-related infections. *Morbidity and Mortality Weekly Report* 51:RR-10.

Chernecky C, Macklin D, Nugent K *et al.* (2002). The need for shared decision making in the selection of vascular access devices: an assessment of patients and clinicians. *Journal of Vascular Access Devices* 7:34–39.

Cole D (1999). Selection and management of central venous access devices in the home setting. *Journal of Intravenous Nursing* 22:315–319.

Cortelezzi A, Frachiolla NS, Maisonneuve P *et al.* (2003). Central venous catheter-related complications in patients with haematological malignancies: a retrospective analysis of risk factors and prophylactic measures. *Leukaemia & Lymphoma* 44:1495–1501.

DOH (Department of Health) (2002). *Reference Guide to Consent for Examination or Treatment*. Department of Health, London, UK.

Dezfulian C, Lavelle J, Nallamouthu BK *et al.* (2003). Rates of infection for single lumen versus multilumen central venous catheters: a meta-analysis. *Critical Care Medicine* 31:2385–2390.

Elliott TSJ, Faroqui MH, Armstrong RF *et al.* (1994). Guidelines for good practice in central venous catheterization. *Journal of Hospital Infection* 28:163–176.

Farkas JC, Liu N, Bleroit JP *et al.* (1992). Single versus triple-lumen central catheter-related sepsis: a prospective randomised study in a critically ill population. *American Journal of Medicine* 93:277–282.

Fletcher SJ, Bodenham AR (1999). Catheter related sepsis: an overview. *British Journal of Intensive Care* 9:46–53.

Gabriel J, Bravery K, Dougherty L *et al.* (2005). Vascular access; indications and implications for patient care. *Nursing Standard* 19:45–54.

Gabriel, J (1999). Long-term central venous access. In *Intravenous Therapy in Nursing Practice*, Dougherty L, Lamb J (eds), Churchill Livingstone, Edinburgh, UK.

Galloway S, Bodenham AR (2004). Long-term central venous access. *British Journal of Anaesthesia* 92:722–734.

Galloway S, Sharma A, Ward J *et al.* (2005). A review of an anaesthetic led vascular access list. *Anaesthesia* 60:772–778.

Goodman M (2000). Chemotherapy: principles of administration. In *Cancer Nursing*, Hanke Yarbro C (ed.), Jones and Bartlett, Sudbiiry, MA, pp. 385–443.

Groeger JS, Lucas AB, Thaler HT *et al.* (1993). Infectious morbidity associated with use of long-term venous access devices in patients with cancer. *Annals of Internal Medicine* 119:1168–1174.

Hamilton H (2000). Selecting the correct IV device: nursing assessment. *British Journal of Nursing* 9:968–978.

Hamilton H, Fermo K (1998). Assessment of patients requiring IV therapy via a central venous route. *British Journal of Nursing* 7:451–460.

Hatfield A, Bodenham AR (1999). Portable ultrasound for difficult venous access. *British Journal of Anaesthesia* 82:822–826.

Henriques HF, Kanny-Jones R, Knoll SM *et al.* (1993). Avoid complications of long-term venous access. *American Surgery* 9:555–558.

Infusion Nurses Society (INS) (2006). Infusion nursing standards of practice. *Journal Intravenous Nursing* 29:S1–S92.

Intravenous Nurses Society (INS) (2000). *Standards for Infusion Therapy*, INS and Becton Dickinson, Cambridge, MA.

Knutsad K, Hager B, Hauser M *et al.* (2003). Radiological diagnosis and management of complications related to central venous access. *Acta Radiologica* 44:508–516.

Maki DG, Crnich CJ (2005). History forgotten, is history relived: nosocomial infection control is also essential in the outpatient setting. *Archives Internal Medicine* 165:2565–2567.

Mermel LA, McCormack RD, Springman SR *et al.* (1991). The pathogenesis and epidemiology of catheter-related infection with pulmonary artery Swan-Ganz catheters: a prospective study using molecular sub-typing. *American Journal of Medicine* 91:S197–S205.

NICE (2002). *Guidance on the use of ultrasound locating devices for central venous catheters* (NICE technology appraisal, No. 49.), London. Available at www.nice.org.

NICE (2003). *Infection Control: Prevention of Healthcare Associated Infection in Primary and Community Care*, Clinical guideline CG2, London. Available at www.nice.org.

Pegues D, Axelrod P, McClarren C *et al.* (1992). Comparison of infections in Hickman and implanted port catheters in adult solid tumor patients. *Journal of Surgical Oncology* 49:156–162.

Pratt RJ, Pellow C, Loveday H *et al.* (2001). The epic project: developing evidence-based guidelines for the prevention of healthcare associated infections. *Journal of Hospital Infection* 47:S1–S82.

Raad II, Hohn DC, Gilbreath BJ *et al.* (1994). Prevention of central venous catheter-related infections by using maximal sterile barrier precautions during insertion. *Infection Control and Hospital Epidemiology* 15:231–238.

Randolph AG, Cook DJ, Gonzales CA *et al.* (1998). Tunnelling short-term central venous catheters to prevent catheter-related infection: a meta-analysis of randomised controlled trials. *Critical Care Medicine* 26:1452–1455.

RCN (Royal College of Nursing Intravenous Therapy Forum) (2005). RCN standards for infusion therapy. *Royal College of Nursing*, London, UK.

Royal College of Anaesthetists (2001). Implementing and ensuring safe sedation practice for healthcare procedures in adults. Report of an Intercollegiate Working Party. Available at www.rcoa.ac.uk.

Sansivero GE (1998). Venous anatomy and physiology. Considerations for vascular access device placement and function. *Journal of Intravenous Nursing* 21:S107–S114.

Veseley TM (2003). Central venous catheter tip: a continuing controversy. *Journal of Intravascular and Interventional Radiology* 14:527–534.

Whitman ED (1996). Complications associated with the use of central venous access devices. *Current Problems in Surgery* 23:309–388.

Chapter 4

Catheter design and materials

Fiona Ives

Introduction

In the last few years, there has been a considerable increase in the numbers and varieties of central venous access devices (CVADs) inserted. These are used in a variety of ways, both for short-term and long-term use (Vazquez 2005). Operators need to understand the differences between such devices in order to make an informed choice of catheter. Procedures such as haemodialysis and apheresis require a totally different kind of CVAD, compared to one used for the administration of antibiotics, cytotoxic drugs or parenteral nutrition. Clinical aspects of patient assessment and catheter selection are covered in Chapter 3.

Several factors must be taken into consideration when individually assessing the patient and recommending which CVAD should be used. Standardising the types of CVAD used in each institution is beneficial, as this will assist both the staff inserting the CVAD and subsequent users to become familiar with a product (Hamilton 2000). This can help in reducing complications associated with CVADs, e.g. thrombus formation. If the catheter material is of a low thrombotic formulation, and the right size for the chosen vein, this will reduce the risk of thrombus and stenosis.

Material differences

Polyurethane CVADs are biocompatible with most drugs and are resistant to many chemicals. However, the use of alcohol-based cleaning agents may weaken or perish the catheter. This material is thromboresistant and will soften within the body, therefore reducing mechanical trauma and irritation within the vein compared to harder materials. Another advantage of polyurethane is its tensile strength, permitting the manufacturers of these catheters to develop devices with thinner walls, multiple lumens and smaller external diameters, thereby maximising blood flow within a vessel housing a CVAD (Hadaway 1995, Bard 2000, Vesley 2005). Modern polyurethane catheters are now available as semi-rigid and flexible materials, often used for short-term central venous access. Whilst sufficiently stiff for percutaneous insertion over a wire without a splitting sheath, polyurethane will soften after insertion in response to body temperature, making the device more compliant once positioned within a vein.

Silicone is a soft, pliable, thromboresistant material and is advantageous for catheter construction because of its kink resistance. It is also biocompatible with most drugs. However silicone has a limited tensile strength and can rupture, and so requires restricted infusion flow pressures. It requires insertion through a sheath or cannula. Silicone is compatible with alcohol-based cleaning solutions, but can be degraded by peroxide and some povidone-iodine solutions.

Other types of materials have been used to make CVADs such as PVC, Teflon and polyethylene. These, however, have been replaced in most cases by more sophisticated materials such as polyurethane and silicone.

Thrombosis: the relative risks between materials

Damage to the wall of a vein is related to the stiffness of the catheter (Indar 1959). Polyurethane and PVC were both used in the past due to their stiff nature, which permitted easier percutaneous insertion. However, both materials are associated with increased thrombogenicity due to their rigidity, resulting in damage to the intima of the vein and subsequent platelet aggregation. Whilst catheter stiffness is important, it is possible that the chemical composition is a more significant risk for thrombosis (Ng 1992). A comparison of equally soft polyurethane and silicone catheters (Linder *et al.* 1984) showed that thrombophlebitis occurred significantly less frequently with polyurethane catheters. Earlier studies demonstrated a wide range of thrombogenicity between varying materials. Polyethylene, polypropylene, PVC or nylon catheters all had a tendency to initiate thrombosis if used for long-term use. Hydromer-coated polyurethane performed the best, followed by silicone elastomer (Borow 1985). The most common material currently used for long-term, skin-tunnelled catheters is silicone for its flexibility and low thrombogenicity (Davidson and Al Mufti 1997).

Infection

An important consideration when selecting catheter material is that bacteria adhere to and multiply on the surface of all catheters. Although the surface of a catheter may appear smooth on visual inspection, under electron microscopy the surface resemble lunar craters (Dougherty 2006). Fibrin and bacteria adhere readily to such surfaces resulting in an increased attachment of microorganisms and predispose to thrombus, which in turn may promote bacterial colonisation. Bacterial adherence varies considerably with the type of catheter material (Elliott 1998) (see Chapter 13). Other initiatives have included the redesign of catheter components, formation of new coatings and polymers with less plasticisers and a smoother surface. Various anti-adhesive coatings have also been developed which include hydromers which have been used to coat catheters (Tebbs 1994).

After CVAD insertion, within seconds, platelets interact with the catheter surface, resulting in the catheter becoming coated with body fluids and proteins, with subsequent platelet and fibrin disposition. This process occurs on all foreign substances introduced into the vascular system, although it is more apparent with some materials than others. Due to platelet adhesion and activation, catheters become encased by fibrin within 5–7 days, which in time will develop into a fibrin sheath. Fibrin deposition occurs from the area where the catheter enters the skin to where its tip touches the intima of the vein (Vesely 2003). Improving catheter material by enhancing biocompatibility within a vein, e.g. hydrometric coated catheters as well as bonding catheters with heparin may aid in the reduction of thrombogenicity (Evans Orr 1993).

Some catheters may have antibiotic bonding (e.g. minocycline/rifampin) (Raad 1997), silver impregnation (Modak 1992, Logghe 1997, Maki 1997, Veenestra *et al.* 1999, Schierholz 2000, Crnich 2004) to the entire length of the device, providing protection against potential bacteria seeding to the catheter. Other devices are bonded with antiseptic material, such as silver sulfadiazine and chlorhexidine. These designs have been marketed with claims of a reduction in colonisation and infection rates, although more research is needed to prove their efficacy and cost-effectiveness in different patient groups.

The majority of studies on this subject have been conducted using non-cuffed multiple lumen catheters on adult patients in a critical care setting, which have remained in situ for less than 30 days. The benefits have been well established, and they are recommended for use in high-risk areas such as critical care where infection rates are high (DOH 2001, CDC 2002). Other devices are now available for longer-term use, e.g. silver impregnated cuffed tunnelled catheters (Vygon), but their longer-term efficacy is as yet unproven.

All these catheter coatings have risks in terms of patient sensitivity to the drug coating or the emergence of bacterial resistance in the case of antimicrobials.

Catheter design

Catheters are designed in many different varieties and the advantages and disadvantages or each should be kept in mind when assessing the patient and recommending which CVAD is the best choice. The design of the catheter will dictate insertion techniques, which include the catheter being passed over needle, through needle, over a guidewire or through a sheath.

Tip design

There are multiple tip shapes found in central venous catheters (Figure 4.1).

Open-ended non-tapered: Single, double or triple lumen catheters are available that open directly out at the end, which can be cut to meet the needs of individual patient, in terms of length and position. Examples are Hickman and PICC soft silicone-type catheters. Such soft blunt-tipped devices will generally require to be inserted through a sheath or catheter into the vein.

Open-ended tapered: Such catheters are of fixed length and cannot be cut. The tapered tip allows passage over guidewires or needles if the catheter is stiff enough. Multilumen catheters will generally have staggered openings, often with a soft atraumatic tip.

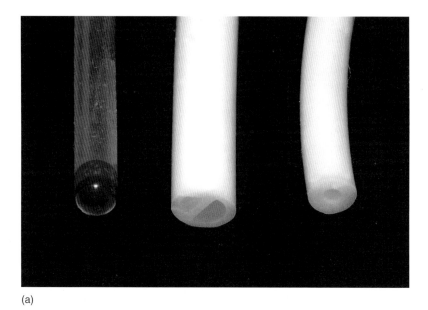

(a)

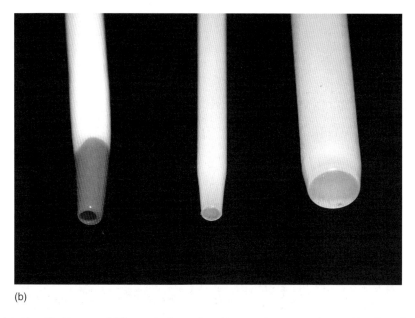

(b)

Figure 4.1 Magnified images of different tip shapes found in central venous catheters. (a) Left: preformed tip of Groschong catheter, middle: double lumen (9.5 fr) Hickman catheter which is cut to length by operator, right: cut end of silicone port catheter. Note relatively thick walls due to low tensile strength of silicone. All are inserted through a peel away sheath. (b) Left: preformed soft tip of multiple lumen catheter (as shown in Figure 4.6) inserted over a guidewire, middle: tip of catheter over needle device (as in Figure 4.3), right: tip of introducer sheath (Figure 4.7 upper) inserted over an obturator. All thin-walled polyurethane devices.

Open-ended catheters will develop blood reflux which will clot and cause catheter blockage if the device is not flushed regularly and effectively. This problem increases as the bore of the device increases (see Chapter 14). Such reflux can be reduced by the use of devices where the catheter tip is valved, as in Groshong catheters. There are also catheters available with the valve within the proximal hub of the catheter (see below).

Insertion techniques

The guidewire or Seldinger (1953) technique

This begins with a needle being introduced into a vein; a guidewire is then passed through the needle. After the removal of the needle, the catheter is introduced into the vein over the guidewire. One or more dilators may be required to enlarge the tract prior to catheter insertion. A modification of this technique involves the use of a tapered vein dilator with a sheath, through which catheters can be inserted (Ng 1992).

The advantage of such techniques is that the vein can be accessed with a small-bore needle and the use of a guidewire greatly increases the success of central passage of soft flexible catheters. The technique can be further refined using very fine needles and guidewires to access the vein and then dilate the tract to accommodate larger devices, so-called micropuncture techniques (Figure 4.2).

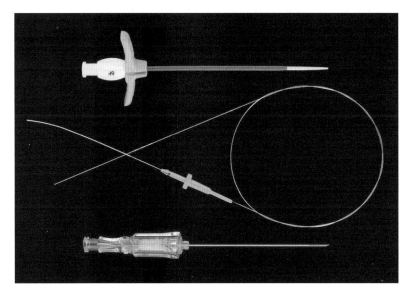

Figure 4.2 Micropuncture needle and guidewire. Microaccess kit Vygon, UK. The fine bore needle 21 g with needle guard system is used to gain access to a small or large vessel and the fine bore coated guidewire inserted. The tract is then dilated to accommodate larger catheters via the 5-Fr dilator and splitting sheath. Such kit improves success and safety in catheterisation in the more challenging case.

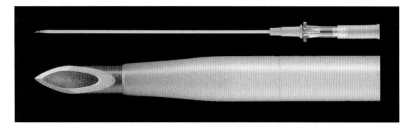

Figure 4.3 A catheter over needle device. A 16 g 5-in. long angiocath device (upper) (Becton Dickinson). Close-up of tip design (lower).

Catheter over needle devices

This design was developed to eliminate the risk of the needle cutting through the catheter during the insertion process. The needle lies within the catheter and both are inserted together when the vein is punctured (Figure 4.3) (Hoffer *et al*. 1999). The needle is then withdrawn and the catheter advanced along the vein. One advantage of this technique is that the hole made in the vein by the needle is smaller than the actual size of the catheter. Therefore, leakage of blood is less likely than catheters inserted using catheter through the needle devices. Such devices are limited by the requirement for the needle to be the same bore as the catheter, the practical length of the needle and the presence of a single lumen only. Such devices are in routine use for peripheral cannulation, but have been largely superseded by Seldinger-based techniques for CVADs in most centres.

Catheter through needle/cannula

Puncture of the vein is performed using a short cannula with the needle inside. The needle is withdrawn and the soft flexible catheter is inserted through the cannula (Ng 1992). Such devices are designed for both short-term (Figure 4.4) and longer use (see discussion on PICCs below). Disadvantages of this technique remain. It is possible that the cannula tip does not reside within the lumen of the vein. In addition, the catheter is smaller than the hole in the vein, and therefore it is possible that blood may leak around the catheter. Catheters through needle techniques run the risk of cutting the catheter and have been largely superseded.

Needle design

Standard 18 or 19 g needles are used in most adult central venous access sets. Some manufacturers' needles are considerably sharper than others, and relatively blunt needles make accessing the vein difficult. Needle tips blunt quickly with use. If difficulties are experienced in puncturing the skin, or the vein is seen to be repeatedly collapse on ultrasound imaging as the needle approaches it, consider the use of new sharp needle. Small collapsible veins may be accessed more easily with a micropuncture needle and

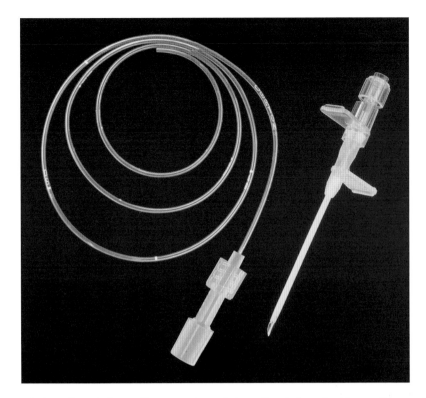

Figure 4.4 Catheter through the needle or cannulae technique. Cavafix 'long line' Braun, Germany. The 16 g 70-cm long catheter (shown coiled) is passed via the 14 g short intravenous cannula into a large arm vein and advanced centrally to place the tip in the SVC. There is a long removable plastic stiffener within the catheter. Such devices are typically used for short-term central venous access during anaesthesia and surgery.

guidewire (Figure 4.2). The increasing interest in ultrasound guidance means that many kits now have needles with machined tips to increase visibility under ultrasound (see Chapter 9), but their overall value is debated. Some operators prefer to use a needle and cannula for initial access to the vein, the guidewire is then introduced through the cannula rather than the needle.

Catheter size

Catheter size will depend on the patient assessment and the treatment required. Small-bore catheters will be adequate for intermittent or slow infusion of drugs, but will not allow rapid infusion of blood and other fluids. Manufacturers typically provide tables of approximate flow rates for 0.9% saline (not more viscid blood products), for a given catheter size which is a function of lumen size and length. Multiple lumens are required for simultaneous infusion of incompatible products. Smaller sizes of dilators, sheaths and catheters should reduce the risk of vessel damage during insertion and are more

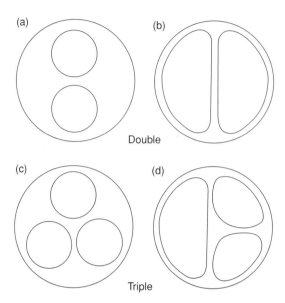

(a)

(b)

Double

(c)

(d)

Triple

Figure 4.5 Cross section of two double lumen catheters (a and b), and two triple lumen catheters (c and d) showing different arrangements of lumens (Ng 1992).

likely to traverse corners without the use of excessive force. See Chapter 11 for insertion tips for such devices.

Multilumen catheters

A multilumen catheter is a CVAD with more than one channel, these channels being separated by a thin wall preventing mixing of infusates (Figures 4.5 and 4.6). The number of lumens can range from one to five. The lumen diameter will determine the flow rate through the catheter. Use the smallest number of lumens possible, as they all represent a cumulative infection risk (see Chapter 13). There are dangers of mixing infusates if a fibrin sleeve develops, and extravasation injury is possible if the proximal exit hole lies in subcutaneous tissue due to outward migration of catheter.

Common types of catheters

Acute care catheter

This catheter is usually composed of polyurethane and is typically used in acute cases where short-term access is required, e.g. major surgery, critical care and accident and emergency. It is typically a relatively short-tapered open-ended multilumen catheter (Figure 4.6) and can be used for 3–10 days or longer (depending on local institutional guidelines). A range of different fixed length will be required for each route of access,

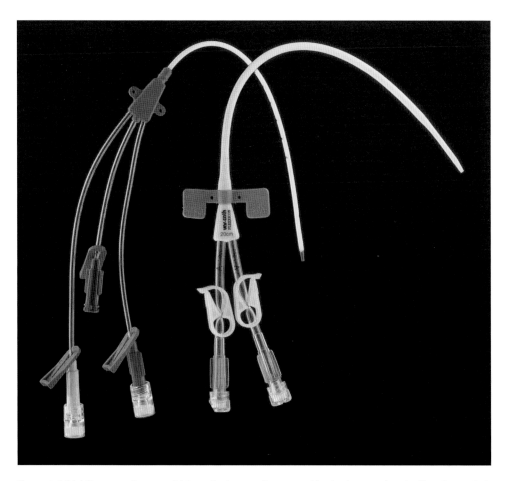

Figure 4.6 Multilumen catheters, which are both passed over a guidewire into an already dilated tract. Left: triple lumen 7 Fr × 16 cm multiplex catheter (Smiths, Germany) typically used in anaesthesia, surgery and acute care for short-term central venous access. Right: widebore dual lumen non-cuffed Vas-Cath short-term dialysis/apheresis catheter with a staggered distal lumen exits holes at the tip to avoid recirculation of blood.

e.g. right internal jugular 12–15 cm, left internal jugular 15–18 cm, right subclavian 18–20 cm, left subclavian 22–26 cm, femoral 25–30 cm.

Introducer sheaths

These are in widespread use for introduction of many different devices into the circulation and come in a very wide range of sizes and lengths. Valve arrangements (Figure 4.7) allows devices to be passed in and out without bleeding or air entry, and allow intermittent insertion or manipulation of catheters in and out of the vein, e.g. a pulmonary artery catheter or pacing wire. Splitting sheaths (Figure 4.7) enable removal of the sheath without it passing over the device to be inserted, e.g. during Hickman line insertion procedures.

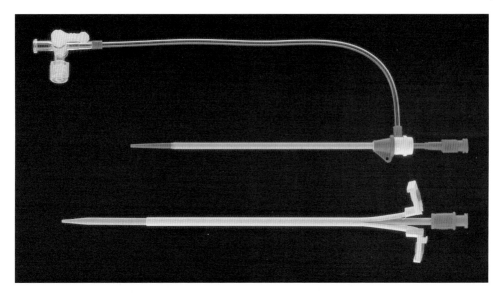

Figure 4.7 Upper: 8-Fr multipurpose introducer valved sheath with side arm and dilator/introducer, Cordis, USA. Once inserted over a guidewire into a blood vessel, this device can be used to introduce and manipulate guidewires, pacing wires, cardiac catheters and other devices. Fluids can be injected via the sidearm. Lower: 11-Fr splitting (peel away) sheath and dilator/introducer (Vygon, UK). Once inserted into a blood vessel over a guidewire, intravascular devices (e.g. a Hickman catheter) can be inserted through the sheath which is then split apart to allow it to be removed, without passing over the inserted device.

Midline catheters

These catheters have a limited duration of 2–4 weeks. They are predominantly composed of silicone and are inserted via the veins around the antecubital fossa (Figure 4.8). They are designed so that the tip is situated in the basilic or cephalic vein below the axillary vein. Single and dual lumen catheters are available. They are typically inserted via a short-length cannula or a splitting sheath. Typical flow rates are shown in Table 4.1.

Peripherally inserted central catheters

PICCs can be made of polyurethane or silicone and come in many forms depending on the supplier including those with single, dual or triple lumens. They are inserted via the antecubital fossa or upper arm with catheter tip placement ideally in the lower SVC. They are recommended for mid-term therapy from 6 weeks to 1 year (Bard 2000). They are typically inserted via a needle and cannula or short guidewire and splitting sheath. Some are passed over a long guidewire to a central position (see Chapter 8).

PICCs can be valved (Figure 4.9) or non-valved. The latter is open-ended and will have a clamp to stop flow through its lumen. It requires regular positive flushing after every use to prevent blood back flow, which will occlude the catheter. Valved PICCs

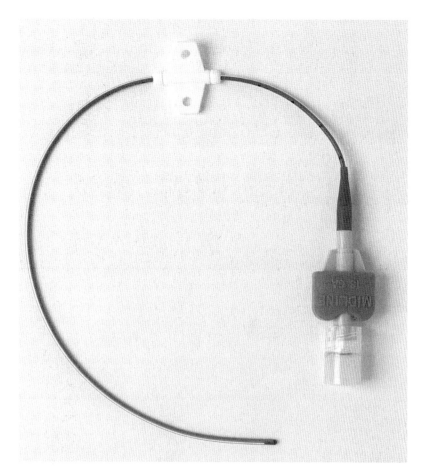

Figure 4.8 A midline catheter with detachable suture wing (Bard USA). This has a preformed Groshong valve tip.

(Groshong) incorporate a pressure-sensitive valve at the side of the distal end that allows fluid infusion and blood aspiration. When not in use, the valve restricts blood back flow and air embolism. Such valves mean that heparinised flushes are not required. Typical flow rates are shown in Table 4.2.

Table 4.1 Midline catheter flow rates.

	Single lumen				Dual lumen	
Catheter size Fr	3	4	5	6	5	6
Lumen size (mm)	0.6	0.8	1	1.2	0.7	0.8
Flow millilitre per hour (0.9% saline)	400	1220	1500	1900	350	350

All flows relate to gravity flow for normal saline at 1m head height.
Data from Bard USA.

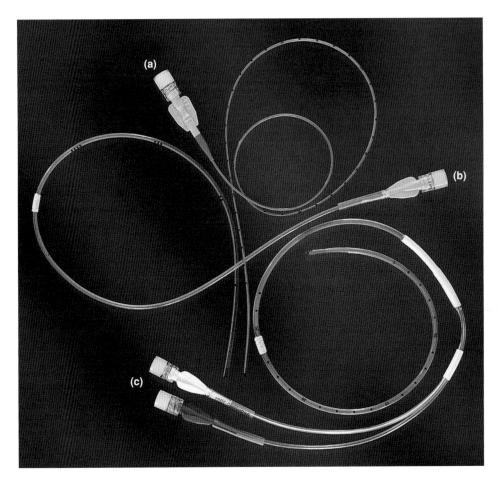

Figure 4.9 Three catheters with Groshong valved tips (Bard USA). A, A single lumen PICC, B, a single lumen cuffed catheter. C, a double lumen cuffed catheter.

Table 4.2 PICC flow rates.

	Single lumen				Dual lumen	
Catheter size Fr	3	4	5	6	5	6
Lumen size (mm)	0.6	0.8	1	1.2	0.7	0.7
Flow millilitre per hour (0.9% saline)	100	400	800	1300	150	400

All flows relate to gravity flow for normal saline at 1m head height.
Data from Bard USA.
Note: Flow rate will increase if the catheter is cut to shorter length.

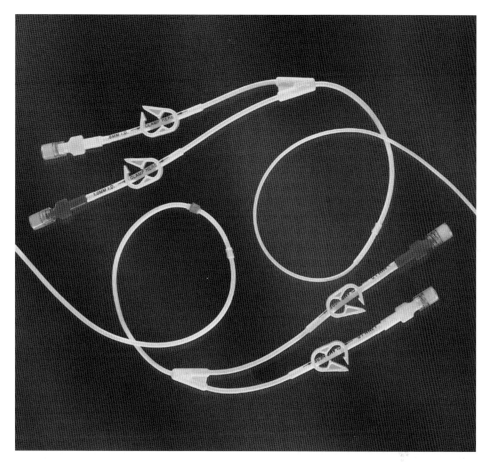

Figure 4.10 Dual lumen open-ended, non-valved Hickman catheters (Bard USA). These have an anchoring Dacron cuff, and one has an additional antimicrobial cuff to be sited near the skin exit site.

Tunnelled cuffed catheters

The tunnelled catheter design has a Dacron cuff, which enables tissue in-growth to anchor the catheter into the subcutaneous tissue. The cuff also acts as a barrier to the spread of microorganisms from the exit site along the external surface of the catheter. The material used for this catheter can be polyurethane or silicone, and it is available with single, dual or triple lumens. Such devices are available in valved and non-valved versions (Figures 4.9 and 4.10). The non-valved variety has an open-ended design with separate clamps on each lumen (Hickman- and Broviac-type catheters). Typical flow rates are shown in Table 4.3.

There are two types of valved catheter. The tunnelled cuffed Groshong catheter is composed of silicone with a Dacron anchoring cuff with valve at the side of the distal tip (Figure 4.11) as with the Groshong PICC. It does not require a clamp or heparin use to maintain patency. It is designed with single and double lumens. The Dacron cuff

Table 4.3 Tunnelled Catheter flow rates.

	Single lumen				Dual lumen				Triple lumen	
Catheter size (Fr)	2.7	4.2	6.6	9.6	7.0	9.0	10	12	10	12.5
Lumen size ID (mm)	0.5	0.7	1.0	1.6	0.8/1.0	0.7/1.3	1.3/1.3	1.6/1.6	1.5/08/0.8	1.5/1.0/1.0
Flow		50	200	500	>500	All>500mls/hour			All>500mls/hour	

All flows relate to gravity flow for normal saline at 1m head height.
Data from Bard USA.

used to anchor this device is rather less bulky than other devices. The valve precludes its use for central vein pressure monitoring and requires pressurised infusion devices to achieve flow, gravity alone is usually insufficient.

The second type of valved catheter is the Boston Scientific Pressure Activated Safety Valve (PASV) catheter, similar in performance to the Groshong valve, the valve automatically resists backflow and generally eliminates the need to use heparin to maintain patency. The PASV valve is designed to be pressure activated and direction specific. For

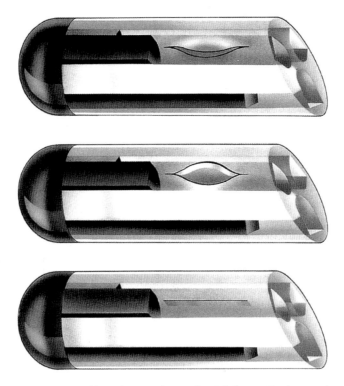

Figure 4.11 (a) Magnified image of the valve near the tip of a triple lumen Groshong catheter (Bard USA). Aspiration of the lumen induces a negative pressure opening the slit valve inwards (upper image). Flushing the device induces a positive pressure opening the slit valve outwards (middle image).

infusion, minimal pressure opens the valve to deliver infusates. It is designed to stay closed as central venous pressure rises. For blood sampling, pressure is achieved by aspiration. The valve is in the proximal hub of the catheter.

Apheresis and Haemodialysis catheters

These are composed of silicone or polyurethane and can be cuffed or non-cuffed dependent on the proposed duration of use. These catheters are large bore and are of relatively stiff construction to avoid wall collapse from the negative pressures from pumped systems. Typically, the lumen has an end hole and multiple side holes to improve flows and mixing of blood. They can be two functionally separate catheters (e.g. Tesio device Figure 4.12) which are inserted in parallel so their tips lie slightly separated in the same vein. Others are a combined dual or triple lumen catheter with a staggered-end design with one lumen positioned 3–5 cm above the other, to prevent recirculation of the treated blood (Figure 4.13). Both lumens have clamps and the catheter tip needs to be placed in the lower SVC, right atrium or the IVC rather than more peripherally to achieve good blood flows. To prevent thrombotic events occurring within this type of catheter, heparin locks are essential if patency is to be assured. Late catheter malfunction is often the consequence of fibrin deposition around the catheter tip – an unpredictable process but one that occurs more frequently in some and less frequently in others (Moss *et al.* 1990, McDowell *et al.* 1993).

Totally implanted ports

The design of ports enables a tunnelled catheter to end in a reservoir, which has been implanted subcutaneously (Figures 4.14 and 4.15). The reservoir has a thick self-sealing silicone diaphragm accessible by percutaneous puncture with a special non-coring needle (Figure 4.16). Ports are available with different sizes of catheters attached to single or dual lumen reservoir (one reservoir per lumen) in high- or low-profile design. The port can be made of titanium or plastic, and if the patient needs frequent MRI scans, plastic ports should be used. Ports are ideal for intermittent injections so the needle is not in situ for long time periods. They have the lowest risk of catheter-related sepsis due to the intact skin barrier. They are expensive compared to other long-term access devices and require increased surgical time to insert and remove.

Anchorage devices

Securing a central venous access device is vital if complications related to poor tip position, extravasation and total dislodgement are to be prevented (see Chapter 12).
   Securement can be achieved in various ways:

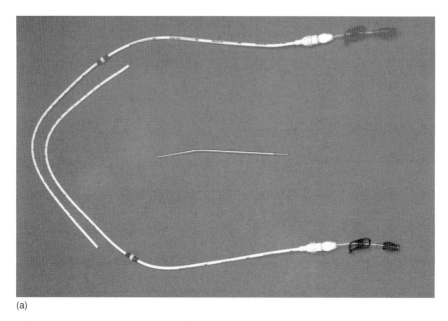

(a)

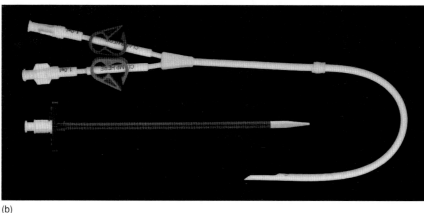

(b)

Figure 4.12 (a) Tesio catheter for long-term dialysis/apheresis consisting of two separate silicone-cuffed tunnelled catheters which are inserted side by side usually via the right internal jugular with their tips slightly separated to prevent blood recirculation (Medcomp USA). Different lengths will be required for each route of access due to its fixed length. The cuff is in two parts; bulky plastic to provide some immediate mechanical anchorage plus a Dacron sleeve to provide longer-term anchorage. A small tunnelling rod is also shown.
(b) Vygon 14-Fr dual lumen apheresis/dialysis cuffed catheter with introducer and splitting sheaths. Different lengths will be required for each route of access due to its fixed length.

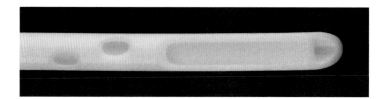

Figure 4.13 Tip of dual lumen 14-Fr apheresis catheter (Vygon, UK) (see whole device in Figure 4.12). The two lumens are separated by approximately 3 cm to avoid recirculation of treated blood.

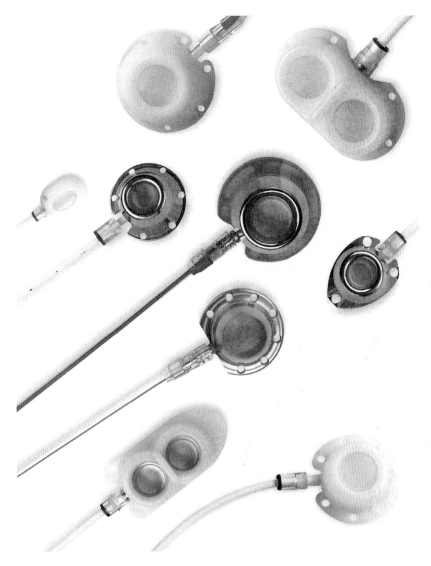

Figure 4.14 Single and dual lumen high- and low-profile ports (Bard USA). Such devices can be made of titanium or plastic (MRI compatible).

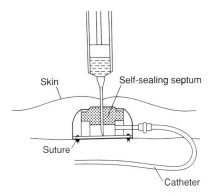

Figure 4.15 Cross-sectional diagram of a port in situ showing needle access to a port (Hamilton 2000).

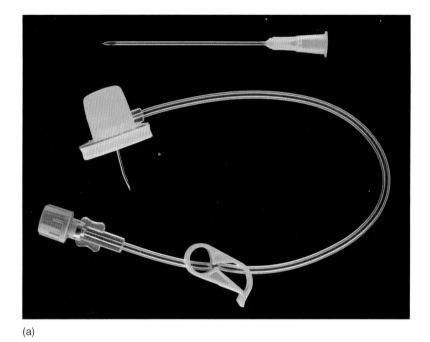

(a)

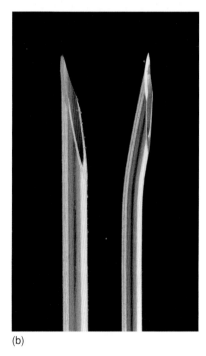

(b)

Figure 4.16 Non-coring Huber needle designed to gain access via a port. (a) 'Gripper portacath' needle 20 g 19 mm long (SIMS, USA) designed with non-coring tip for accessing vascular ports with standard 19 g white needle for comparison. (b) Tips of same needles magnified to show standard cutting and non-coring tip (right).

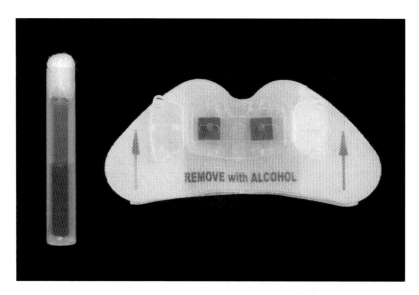

Figure 4.17 Statlock catheter securement device and adhesive solution applicator (left) (Bard USA). The adhesive anchoring device replaces sutured anchor wings for skin fixation of vascular catheters.

- Adhesive sterile dressings are available in a wide range of sizes and materials (see Chapter 14).
- The majority of non-tunnelled central venous catheters are designed with suture holes, in fixed or detachable suture wings. Such sutures are effective but are difficult to clean around, enhance local infection, and are uncomfortable for the patient.
- Skin-tunnelled CVADs were traditionally secured by suturing through the skin and tying the sutures around the catheter. There is a risk of damage to catheters when such sutures are removed. Alternatively, newer devices have detachable suture wings. Such sutures should remain in situ until the Dacron cuff is fixed in subcutaneous tissues. This process takes at least 2–3 weeks.
- Specific securing devices, such as the 'Statlock' (Yamamoto 2002, Schears 2005) (Figure 4.17), which are designed purely for securing CVADs, are available reducing the risk of migration with a lower incidence of infection during their use (Stacey 2000).

Conclusion

The eclectic selection of CVADs available on the market, added to the different requirements of each patient can cause confusion and inappropriate selection of devices. Optimal results are obtained by using the most appropriate central venous access device that will accomplish the intended treatment plan.

References

Bard CR (2000). Accessibility. www.accessabilitybybard.co.uk.

Borow M, Crowley JG (1985). Evaluation of central venous catheter thrombogenicity. *Acta Anaesthesiologia Scandinavica* S81:59.

CDC (Center for Disease Control) (2002). Guidelines for the prevention of intravascular catheter related infections. *Morbidity and Mortality Weekly Report*, Vol. 51, pp. 1–26.

Crnich CJ, Maki DG (2004). Are antimicrobial-impregnated catheters effective? Don't throw the baby out with the bathwater. *Clinical Infectious Diseases* 38:1287–1292.

Davidson T, Al Mufti R (1997). Hickman central venous catheters in cancer patients. *Cancer Topics* 10:10–14.

DOH (Department of Health) (2001). Guidelines for preventing infections associated with the insertion and maintenance of central venous catheters. *Journal of Hospital Infection* 47:S47–S67.

Dougherty L (2006). *Central Venous Access Devices*, Blackwell Publishing, Oxford, pp. 18–19.

Elliott TSJ (1998). Prevention of central venous catheter related infection. *Journal of Hospital Infection* 40:193–201.

Evans Orr M (1993). Issues in management of peripheral central venous catheters. *Nursing Clinics of North America* 28:911–918.

Hadaway LC (1995). Comparison of vascular access devices. *Seminars in Oncology Nursing* 11:154–166.

Hamilton H (2000). *Total Parenteral Nutrition. A Practical Guide for Nurses.* Churchill Livingstone, Edinborough, UK.

Hoffer EK, Borsa J, Santulli P *et al.* (1999). Prospective randomized comparison of valved versus nonvalved peripherally inserted central vein catheters. *American Journal of Roentgenology* 173:1393–1398.

Indar R (1959). The danger of indwelling polyethylene cannulae in deep veins. *Lancet* 1:284.

Linder L, Curelaru I, Gustavsson B *et al.* (1984). Material thrombogenicity in central venous catheterization: a comparison between soft, antebrachial catheters of silicone elastomer and polyurethane. *Journal of Parenteral and Enteral Nutrition* 8:39.

Logghe C, Van Ossel C, D'Hoore W *et al.* (1997). Evaluation of chlorhexadine and silver-sulfadiazone impreginated central venous catheters for the prevention of bloodstream infection in leukaemic patients: a randomised controlled trial. *Journal or Hospital Infection* 37:145–146.

Maki DG, Stolzs S, Wheeler S *et al.* (1997). Prevention of central venous catheter related blood-stream infection by the use of an antiseptic impregnated catheter – a radomised control trial. *Annals of Internal Medicine* 127:257–266.

McDowell DE, Moss AH, Vasilakis C *et al.* (1993). Percutaneously placed dual lumen silicone catheters for long term use. *American Surgeon* 59:569–573.

Modak SM, Sampath L (1992). Development and evaluation of a new polyurethane central venous antiseptic catheter: reducing central venous catheter infections. Complications in Surgery 11:23–28.

Moss AH, Vasilakis C, Holley JL *et al.* (1990). Use of a silicone dual lumen catheter with a Dacron cuff as a long term vascular access for haemodialysis. *American Journal of Kidney Diseases* 16:211–215.

Ng S (2000). Choosing the equipment. In *Percutaneous Central Venous and Arterial Catheterisation*. Latto IP, NG WS, Jones PL, Jenkins B (eds), 3rd edn. WB Saunders London, UK, pp. 13–31.

Raad I Darouiche R, Dupuis J *et al.* (1997). Central venous catheters coated with minocycline and rifampacin for the prevention of catheter related colonization and bloodstream infections. A randomized double blind trial. *Annals of Internal Medicine* 127:267–274.

Schears GJ (2005). The benefits of a catheter securement device on reducing patient complications. *Managing Hospital Infection* 5:14–20.

Schierholz JM, Fleck C, Beuth J *et al.* (2000). The antimicrobial efficacy of a new central venous catheter with long term broad spectrum activity. *Journal of Antimicrobial Chemotherapy* 46:45–50.

Seldinger SI (1953). Catheter replacement of needle in percutaneous arteriography: new technique. *Acta Radiologica* 39:368.

Stacey W (2000). Teddy holds fast. A nurse-led audit of statlock anchoring devices. Poster presented at NAVAN Conference San Diego, CA, September.

Tebbs SE, Elliott TSJ (1994). Modifications of central venous catheter polymers to prevent in-vitro microbial colonisation. *European Journal of Clinical Microbiology Infection Disease* 13:111–117.

Vazquez MA (2005). The tunnelled catheter is a mature technology and a commercial commodity. *Journal of Vascular Access* 6:137.

Veenestra DL, Saint S, Saha S *et al.* (1999). Efficacy of antiseptic impregnated central venous catheters in preventing catheter related bloodstream infection. *JAMA* 281:261–267.

Vesely TM (2003). Central venous catheter tip position: a continuing controversy. *Journal of Cardiovascular and Interventional Radiology* 14:527–534.

Vesley TM (2005). Tunnelled catheter design: does it matter? *Journal of Vascular Access* 6:132–37.

Yamamoto AJ, Solomon JA, Soulen MC *et al.* (2002). Sutureless securement device reduces complications of peripherally inserted central venous catheters. *Journal of Vascular and Interventional Radiology* 13:77–81.

Chapter 5

Cannulation of the jugular veins

Catherine Farrow, Andrew R. Bodenham and Julian Millo

Introduction

Since the original description of a large series of internal jugular vein (IJV) cannulations (English *et al.* 1969a,b), this route has remained a popular choice for short- and longer-term cannulation. This chapter describes the relevant anatomy and more general considerations for cannulation of both the IJV and external jugular vein (EJV), with an overview of the technique itself. Specific challenges and potential complications are also discussed.

The internal jugular vein

The IJV can be used as a route of access for any part of the systemic venous system. It is chosen because it is large superficial vein that has reasonably consistent surface landmarks and easy ultrasound visualisation, making cannulation generally predictable. In addition, the straight course into the SVC means that devices do not have to traverse corners, and the catheter tip generally passes into the SVC or right atrium, so reducing the requirement for screening during insertion. This also allows the insertion of large-bore and relatively inflexible devices.

Applied anatomy of the IJV

The IJV emerges from the skull through the jugular foramen and runs downwards through the neck in the carotid sheath. It unites with the subclavian vein behind the sternal end of the clavicle to form the brachiocephalic vein (Figure 5.1). Also, in the carotid sheath lies the carotid artery initially anterior then usually medial to the vein and the vagus nerve. The most important relations are the internal, external and common carotid arteries medially and the apex of the lung anterolaterally. Other nearby important structures include the phrenic nerve, thyroid lobe, sympathetic chain,

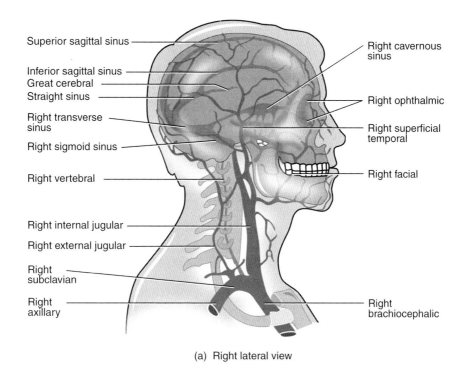

Superior sagittal sinus

Inferior sagittal sinus
Great cerebral
Straight sinus

Right transverse
sinus

Right sigmoid sinus

Right vertebral

Right internal jugular

Right external jugular

Right
subclavian

Right
axillary

Right cavernous
sinus

Right ophthalmic

Right superficial
temporal

Right facial

Right
brachiocephalic

(a) Right lateral view

SUPERIOR

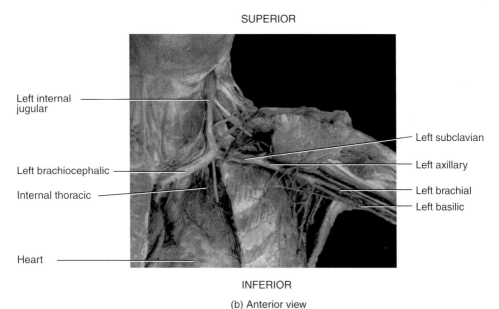

Left internal
jugular

Left brachiocephalic

Internal thoracic

Heart

Left subclavian

Left axillary

Left brachial
Left basilic

INFERIOR

(b) Anterior view

Figure 5.1 (a) Schematic representation of the right sided venous drainage of the head and neck.
(b) Dissection of the left great veins with the clavicle, pectoral muscles and medial aspect of left chest wall
removed. (Both figures from tortora principles of human anatomy).

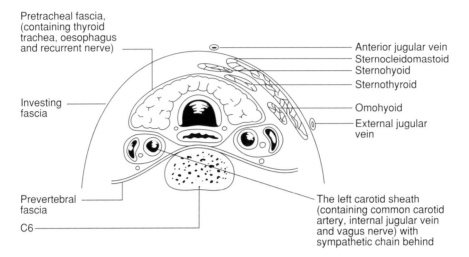

Pretracheal fascia,
(containing thyroid
trachea, oesophagus
and recurrent nerve)

Investing
fascia

Prevertebral
fascia

C6

Anterior jugular vein
Sternocleidomastoid
Sternohyoid
Sternothyroid

Omohyoid
External jugular
vein

The left carotid sheath
(containing common carotid
artery, internal jugular vein
and vagus nerve) with
sympathetic chain behind

Figure 5.2 Cross section of the neck at C6 level (from Ellis' *Anatomy for Anaesthetists* 2004) showing major anatomical structures in relation to internal jugular vein.

vertebral artery, thoracic duct, oesophagus and trachea (Figure 5.2). The vein, artery, thyroid and other structures are easily visualised with ultrasound (Figure 5.3).

The surface markings are a straight line from the mastoid process to the head of the clavicle. The lower part of the IJV lies behind a triangle formed by the junction of the sternal and clavicular insertions of the sternomastoid muscle and the clavicle. The apex of this is used as a surface landmark (Figures 5.4a and 5.4b). Such landmarks are easy to see in the slim patient, but are not visible in the short fat neck (see Chapters 3 and 9).

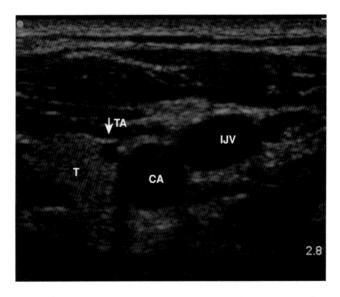

Figure 5.3 Ultrasound cross-sectional image of the right internal jugular vein (IJV) without compression through the probe. Image orientation as seen from the head of the patient. CA, carotid artery; T, thyroid; TA, thyroid artery. Depth of field of image is only 2.8 cm, so all structures are very superficial.

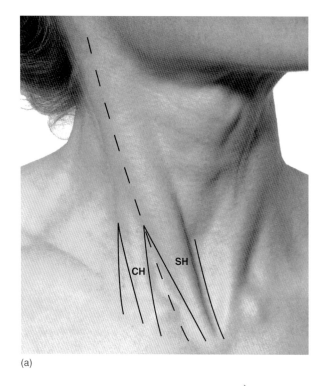

(a)

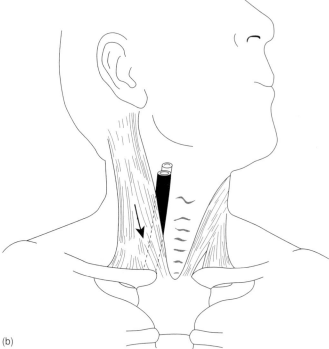

(b)

Figure 5.4 (a) Photograph of right side of neck in a slim female demonstrating surface anatomy. The clavicular (CH) and sternal (SH) heads of sternocleidomastoid are marked. The dashed line indicates the approximate normal course of the internal jugular vein. (b) Diagram showing landmark approaches to the internal jugular vein (from Ellis' *Anatomy for Anaesthetists* 2004). There are a multitude of different approaches described and apparent differences in anatomical relations result from patient variability, neck rotation, flexion/extention of neck, the angle of visualisation (eye or ultrasound) and the level of puncture.

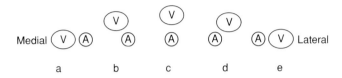

Figure 5.5 Variation in anatomical relations of the right internal jugular vein (V) and common carotid artery (A). a and b rare, c, d, e common. The relationship in e is optimal to avoid inadvertent carotid puncture. See text for further description.

Double transmitted venous pulsations from the heart can be seen in a patient lying down. In heart failure where there is raised venous pressure, this pulsation can be seen in the sitting patient. This is the basis of clinical assessment of the JVP (jugular venous pressure). If the area is pressed down firmly to empty the vein, it will be seen to refill as the vein re-expands. Valves are present, just proximal to where the IJV joins the subclavian vein. The IJV receives multiple tributaries from the pharynx, face, scalp, tongue and thyroid gland. Major lymphatic trunks (the thoracic duct on the left) are present on both the right and left side, with great variability in where they join the venous system. This can be either to the subclavian vein, the IJV or at the junction of the two.

It should be noted that there is significant anatomical variation in the vein and its course as well as in soft tissue neck anatomy. Any pathology of surrounding structures including a goitre or enlarged lymph nodes (see Chapters 3 and 9) will alter the anatomy. The orientation of the vein with respect to the carotid artery is widely variable, in part dependent of the level in the neck. Whilst the vein lies mostly anterolaterally to the artery, a small percentage of patients will have distinctly unfavourable anatomy for surface landmark cannulation, with the vein immediately anterior to the artery or even medial to it (Gordon *et al.* 1998, Dolla 2001, Turba 2005) (Figure 5.5). Commonly, on one side, the vein is larger and more dominant with occasional unilateral congenital absence of the vein. The extensive venous drainage system from the head and neck mean that blockage of the IJV on one side by thrombus or scarring is rarely symptomatic clinically. Although generally straight, the vein may be narrowed, tortuous or absent from congenital or acquired causes (see Figures 5.6 and 5.7). Such variations are easily visualised with ultrasound by scanning from the chosen site of puncture down into the root of the neck to the innominate vein.

Insertion techniques

Numerous landmark-based cannulation techniques, guided by surface landmarks, have been reviewed in detail, along with a thorough description of their advantages and disadvantages (Latto *et al.* 2000). The approaches are broadly divided into so-called high and low approaches, with the high approach arbitrarily defined as being at or above a line drawn level with the cricoid cartilage. The number of approaches is disproportionate to the degree of variation encountered in practice, and evidence suggests that no single route is always reliable and safe (Latto *et al.* 2000). Carotid puncture is unacceptably high in many series and although generally this does not cause problems, occasional severe complications still occur. It is for all the above reasons that ultrasound

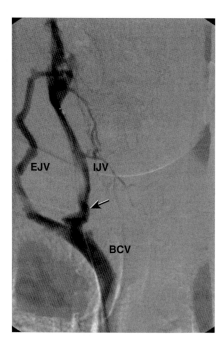

Figure 5.6 A venogram showing a congenital tortuous course (arrow) of the right internal jugular vein (IJV). Similar appearances were also seen in the left neck (not shown). Contrast is also outlining the external jugular vein (EJV). This caused problems with passage of guidewires and cannula after an easy puncture higher in the IJV. It is notable that in this patient, the EJVs were similar in size to the IJVs. BCV, right brachiocephalic vein.

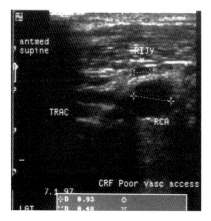

Figure 5.7 A cross-section ultrasound of the left internal jugular and carotid showing a very small vein immediately anterior to the artery. This followed repeated long-term access for dialysis. Such a small vein may represent a narrowed scarred internal jugular vein or a collateral that has opened up following blockage of the main vein.

guidance is now recommended as the preferred method for insertion of central venous catheters into the IJV in adults and children in elective situations (NICE 2002, Karakitos 2006). Furthermore, its use should be considered in most acute clinical circumstances where central venous catheterisation is necessary.

Inexperienced operators need to be supervised. Insertion of a central venous catheter is a practical skill and needs to be taught with graded (decreasing) supervision. It is important to avoid repeated attempts at cannulation and call for experienced assistance appropriately. The technique as described below may need to be adapted in specific circumstances as in the examples described below.

Basic technique for IJV cannulation

Traditionally, the vein has been located by the landmark technique, but the use of ultrasound guidance is now recommended (NICE 2002). Many points of good technique are common to both approaches, to maximise the chances of cannulating the vein and minimise the risk of complications.

Prior to the insertion of a CVC, a detailed clinical assessment should be performed; the procedure explained to the patient and informed consent obtained. Communication with an awake patient should be maintained throughout the procedure. Generous use of local anaesthetic, with or without sedation, is required in an awake patient.

Full aseptic precautions should be employed, including cleaning the skin with 2% chlorhexidine in alcohol. A trained assistant is desirable. The patient should be optimally positioned with a 10° head down tilt (Trendelenburg position) to help distend the vein and reduce the risk of air embolism (Clenaghan *et al.* 2005). If the vein is adequately distended, it is approximately 15 mm in diameter in an adult. A modest degree of rotation of the head away from the side to be cannulated may be necessary, but extreme rotation is best avoided as it may reduce vein diameter. Some head and neck extension is helpful. It is not necessary to place padding under the patient's shoulders.

The equipment should be prepared. The Seldinger technique is the predominant method for direct insertion of catheters into the great veins. The operator stands at the head of the bed. The surface marking of the IJV may be identified by placing the thumb on the mastoid process and the middle finger on the head of the clavicle. The index finger then falls on a point one-third of the way along this line, which is the approximate point of entry for the needle. This point should approximate slightly superior to the apex of the triangle formed by the two heads of the sternocleidomastoid muscle (see Figure 5.4).

The carotid artery can be palpated with the non-dominant hand, adjusting the point of skin entry to be just lateral to the arterial pulse. Excessive pressure by the non-dominant hand should be avoided as this empties the adjacent vein. The position of the vein may be identified with certainty by ultrasound (Figure 5.3), along with the vein diameter, patency and relations to surrounding structures (Hatfield and Bodenham 2005). Some practitioners advocate the use of a small 21G (green) 'seeker' needle to locate the vein, the advantage being that a smaller needle is less likely to cause complications. By using ultrasound, the use of 'seeker' needles may be eliminated.

The cannulation needle will need to be angled downwards at about 30–40°. The needle is directed outwards towards the ipsilateral nipple, avoiding pointing it in a medial direction. Once the position of the carotid artery has been determined, a light touch is all that is required with brief counter traction to allow the needle to pierce the skin. The IJV is superficial in all but the thickest necks, the mean skin to vein distance of the needle being only 2.6 cm in one study comparing 15 different techniques (Metz *et al.* 1984).

Gentle suction should be applied to the needle as it is slowly advanced. A dry syringe is preferable because blood turns bright red when diluted (Ho *et al.* 2000). Recognition that a needle is in the vein should be made by observing the dark colour of venous blood and non-pulsatile nature of the filling of the syringe. If venous blood is not aspirated, it may be that the vein has been transfixed. Apposition of the anterior and posterior walls of the vein frequently occurs, so blood is often only aspirated on withdrawal rather than insertion. The needle should be withdrawn slowly, aspirating gently. When a flashback is seen and venous blood can be aspirated freely, the needle should be kept absolutely still until the guidewire has been successfully threaded. Coating gloved fingers with saline increases the ease with which the wire can be threaded. Ultrasound guidance allows identification of the needle in the IJV and subsequent passage of the guidewire into the chest.

If a guidewire has been passed, and there is concern that it may be in the artery, then a narrow plastic cannula (as supplied in many multiple-lumen central venous catheter kits) can be threaded over the guidewire and connected to a pressure transducer. If the vein is not cannulated, the tip of the needle should be drawn back to just below the skin, where reassessment for the direction for the next pass will be possible. Redirection of the needle whilst in deep tissue is not advised, due to the risk of damage to local structures.

Once the guidewire has been passed, a firm hold of the guidewire should be maintained at all times. The guidewire may have markings to indicate the depth to which it has been inserted. If it is inserted too far, it will irritate the right atrium and cause arrhythmias, most commonly atrial ectopics. Arrhythmias are treated by slight withdrawal of the guidewire.

The guidewire should be checked to ensure free movement by gently moving it in and out of the needle a few centimetres. This action should be repeated after each subsequent step, to check that the guidewire has not become kinked. Should there be any evidence of obstruction as the wire is advanced, no force should be applied.

The needle is slid off the guidewire and a small skin incision made to facilitate dilation of the track. The dilator is passed over the guidewire and the track firmly and smoothly dilated by rotating the dilator between thumb and forefinger as it is advanced. The depth of the vein at cannulation is a guide to how far the dilator needs to be inserted. Care should be taken not to insert the dilator deeper than necessary to minimise the risk of great vein trauma. This is a particular risk if the guidewire has passed into the subclavian vein or other branches, which may not be evident to the operator unless screening is used (Jankovic *et al.* 2005).

When inserting a multiple lumen line, the lumen that opens at the distal tip of the catheter is used to thread the catheter into the vein. It is convenient to prepare the line in advance by priming the other lumens with saline (which may be heparinised) and closing the lumens with three-way taps. Care should be taken not to leave any lumens open to the atmosphere, as this will increase risk of air embolism.

A slightly shorter length of catheter needs to be inserted via the right IJV than the left, typically 15 cm rather than 17 cm. Ideally, the tip should lie outside the right atrium and its position should be checked on a post-procedure chest radiograph.

Specific considerations

Chronic obstructive pulmonary disease

Chronic obstructive pulmonary disease is a common disease of older smokers. Bullae in the apices of the lungs increase the risk of pneumothorax even via the internal jugular route. A higher point of entry is indicated – see Figure 5.4. Ultrasound guidance is recommended.

Hypovolaemic shock

In hypovolaemic shock, the IJV collapses. However, with extreme hypovolaemia, measurement of central venous pressure is not an immediate priority and short, large-bore peripheral cannulae may be a safer initial choice. Ultrasound is useful to identify that the needle has transfixed the vein before withdrawing.

Cardiogenic shock

In cardiogenic shock, central veins are easy to cannulate but the patient may only tolerate lying flat for short periods. Assess vein filling by jugular venous pulse (JVP) or ultrasound and perform the procedure sitting or semirecumbent.

Coagulopathy

Significant coagulopathy is a contraindication to the elective placement of a central venous catheter. Coagulopathy is a common complication of critical illness and a risk/benefit assessment prior to procedures should be made on individual cases. Particular care is needed when the correction of coagulopathy requires the administration of significant volumes of blood products. The routine use of ultrasound will minimise the complications of IJV cannulation (Oquzkurt 2004, 2005, Tercan 2008). The use of the EJV should be considered (see below).

Anatomical variations

The landmark technique for locating the IJV can be compromised by anatomical variability. Individuals with short necks have a smaller distance between the sternal notch and the cricoid cartilage, so there is a higher potential for causing trauma to structures at the root of the neck. Slight extension of the table head may facilitate cannulation.

Vein asymmetry is marked in a small proportion of individuals. Previous cannulation predisposes to thrombosis and stenosis (Raad 1994). The use of ultrasound will identify such abnormalities and aid cannulation.

Other patient factors influencing choice of site

If the patient already has a chest drain in situ, ipsilateral placement would be preferred. Conversely, the side of a known atherosclerotic carotid artery would be avoided because an inadvertent carotid puncture could cause an embolic stroke. Carotid endarterectomy is frequently performed utilising a synthetic Dacron patch to repair the vessel, with attendant risk of graft infection from any catheter-related sepsis (CRS) at this site. In general, such a site should be avoided if possible.

Factors influencing success

Successful cannulation of the IJV requires an appreciation of the relevant anatomy and physiology, training, experience and a confident approach. Failure rates without ultrasound can be as high as 35% (Latto *et al.* 2000). The benefits of ultrasound guidance have been highlighted above (see also Chapter 9) (Randolph *et al.* 1996, Hind *et al.* 2003).

The right IJV is normally slightly larger than the left. Its main advantage is the straight route to the SVC. Most guidewires and catheters will pass blindly into the correct position, and there is considerable leeway for different lengths of catheter and catheter tip position. Large-bore stiff catheters and dilators do not have to traverse tight bends. This is in contrast to catheters passed from the left IJV which have to traverse two corners to get to the SVC and ideal tip position may be problematical unless screening is used (see Chapter 2). The authors recommend use of the right IJV unless other factors dictate an alternate site.

Complications

Whilst the incidence of major complications is low, significant morbidity complicates more than 15% of central venous catheter placements (McGee and Gould 2003). The risks and consequences of complications vary substantially across different patient groups depending on patient anatomy and comorbidities. These complications can be mechanical, infectious or thrombotic. We consider here the complications unique to this route of access (Box 5.1). More general complications are fully discussed in Chapter 12.

Recognised mechanical complications include arterial puncture, bleeding, haematoma, pneumothorax and nerve damage. Less commonly, air embolism, tracheal damage, airway obstruction (from a haematoma) (Figure 5.8), cerebrovascular accident caused by puncture of the vertebral (Figure 5.9) or carotid artery, or loss of guidewire into the central circulation have been reported (Latto *et al.* 2000).

Box 5.1 Complications specific to the IJV route.

Carotid puncture and stroke
Vertebral artery damage and stroke.
Airway obstruction from carotid haematoma
Sympathetic nerve damage (Horner's syndrome)
Tracheal and oesophageal puncture

CRS remains a major problem with a significant mortality rate, despite the use of chlorhexidine-based skin preparation solutions (Maki *et al*. 1991) and/or antiseptic-impregnated central lines. The proximity of the puncture site to oral secretions in the unconscious patient is a problem in critical care. Every catheter should be removed as soon as it is no longer needed, since the probability of CRS increases with time.

Central venous catheterisation predisposes the patient to venous thrombosis and stenosis and can be problematic even in the short-term (Oquzkurt 2004, 2005). A clear relationship exists between this and CRS (Raad 1994).

An acceptable complication rate has never been defined, but interventions to prevent these complications are key (McGee and Gould 2003), particularly the use of ultra-sound (Wigmore 2007). Complication rates are higher in emergency cases and are also associated with duration of placement. Lower rates are seen with experienced personnel (Deshpande *et al*. 2005). Whilst there is evidence to suggest a lower incidence of some mechanical complications compared to the subclavian route, there may be a higher in-cidence of CRS with the internal jugular route (Lorente 2005). More recent studies suggest no statistically significant difference in complications with either approach (Reusch *et al*. 2002, Deshpande *et al*. 2005, Ameh and Jones 2007).

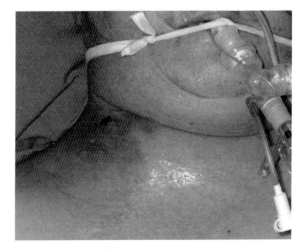

Figure 5.8 Carotid haematoma following attempted right internal jugular catheterisation without ultrasound guidance after thrombolysis and anticoagulation for a myocardial infarction, causing airway obstruction requiring tracheal intubation and assisted ventilation on the intensive care unit.

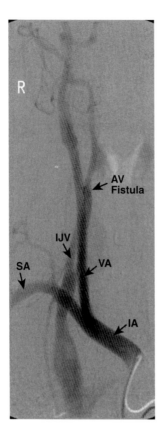

Figure 5.9 Angiogram showing contrast injection up the right innominate (brachiocephalic) artery (IA). Contrast fills the subclavian artery (SA) and vertebral artery (VA). The contrast from the VA refluxes into to the internal jugular vein (IJV) via an AV fistula created after attempted right internal jugular cannulation without ultrasound guidance. The introducing needle simultaneously punctured a venous plexus connected to the jugular vein and the VA close by, to create a fistula. The patient presented with tinnitus in her right ear 6 months later. A bruit could be heard in the neck. The VA was successfully stented radiologically.

The external jugular vein

Introduction

Percutaneous cannulation of the EJV can be used in both adults and children. The EJV is generally easily visible in all but the most obese patients and has the advantages of cannulation under direct vision and ease of application of pressure if haemorrhage occurs. It is particularly useful for rapid access with a standard short intravenous cannula during resuscitation when it usually distended and visible. In suitable cases, a guidewire or catheter can be passed centrally from this route of access.

Applied anatomy

The EJV runs down the neck from the angle of the mandible, before passing over the sternomastoid muscle and penetrating the deep fascia to join the SCV posterior to the clavicle. It is very superficial, contains valves, is mobile and collapses easily. The jaw may obstruct easy needle access along the path of the vein. Its anatomical course makes it difficult or impossible in a significant proportion of patients to pass catheters centrally, as there are multiple sites where obstruction can occur. The vein in many cases takes a tortuous course as it penetrates the cervical fascia to enter deeper layers and in some cases at this site it opens up into multiple branches. Furthermore, there is widespread variation in the size and course of the vein which in some patients may be duplicate or larger than the IJV (see Figure 5.6 of tortuous IJV). It may also drain into the IJV rather than the subclavian vein. Despite these problems, it is a useful route of access, which is often overlooked.

Conclusions

The IJV is a large vein and cannulation is generally predictable and successful. Its proximity to many important structures means that complications are an ever-present risk. The EJV is a useful alternative in some clinical situations. Sound basic technique maximises the chances of success whilst minimising complications. The routine use of real-time, two-dimensional ultrasound needle guidance is recommended for the IJV.

References

Ameh V, Jones S (2007). Central venous catheterisation: internal jugular or subclavian approach? *Emergency Medicine Journal* 24:662–663.

Clenaghan S, McLaughlin RE, Martyn C *et al.* (2005). Relationship between Trendelenburg tilt and internal jugular vein diameter. *Emergency Medicine Journal* 22:867–868.

Deshpande KS, Hatem CC, Ulrich HL *et al.* (2005). The incidence of infectious complications of central venous catheters at the subclavian, internal jugular and femoral sites in an intensive care unit population. *Critical Care Medicine* 33:13–20.

Dolla D, Cavatorta F, Galli S *et al.* (2001). Anatomical variation of internal jugular vein in non-uraemic patients. *Journal of Vascular Access* 2:60–63.

English IC, Frew RM, Pigott JF *et al.* (1969a). Percutaneous cannulation of the internal jugular vein. *Thorax* 24:496–497.

English IC, Frew RM, Pigott JF *et al.* (1969b). Percutaneous catheterisation of the internal jugular vein. *Anaesthesia* 24:521–531.

Gordon, AC, Saliken, JC, Johns D *et al.* (1998). US-guided puncture of the internal jugular vein: complications and anatomic considerations. *Journal of Vascular & Interventional Radiology* 9:333–338.

Hatfield A, Bodenham AR (2005). Ultrasound for central venous access. *Continuing Education in Anaesthesia, Critical Care and Pain* 5:187–190.

Hind D, Calvert N, McWilliams R *et al.* (2003). Ultrasonic locating devices for central venous cannulation: meta-analysis. *BJM* 327:361–364.

Ho AM, Chung DC, Tay BA *et al.* (2000). Diluted venous blood appears arterial: implications for central venous cannulation. *Anesthesia and Analgesia* 91:1356–1357.

Jankovic Z, Boon A, Prasad R *et al.* (2005). Fatal haemothorax following large-bore percutaneous cannulation before liver transplantation. *British Journal of Anaesthesia* 95:472–476.

Karakitos D Labropoulos N, De Groot E *et al.* (2006). Real-time ultra-sound guided catheterisation of the internal jugular vein: a prospective comparison with the landmark technique in critical care patients. *Critical Care* 10:e175.

Latto IP (2000). The internal jugular vein. In *Percutaneous Central Venous and Arterial Catheterisation*, 3rd edn, Latto IP, Ng WS, Jones PL *et al.* (eds), WB Saunders, London, UK, pp. 135–195.

Lorente L, Henry C, Martín MM *et al.* (2005). Central venous catheter-related infection in a prospective and observational study of 2596 catheters. *Critical Care Medicine* 9:R631–R635.

Maki DG, Ringer M, Alvarado CJ *et al.* (1991). Prospective randomised trial of povidone-iodine, alcohol, and chlorhexidine for prevention of infection associated with central venous and arterial catheters. *Lancet* 338:339–343.

McGee DC, Gould MK (2003). Preventing complications of central venous catheterization. *New England Journal of Medicine* 348:1123–1133.

Metz S, Horrow JC, Balcar I *et al.* (1984). A controlled comparison of techniques for locating the internal jugular vein using ultrasonography. *Anesthesia and Analgesia* 63:673.

NICE (National Institute for Clinical Excellence) (2002). Guidance on the use of ultrasound locating devices for placing central venous catheters. *Technology Appraisal Guidance No.49.* Available at www.nice.org.

Oquzkurt L, Tercan F, Torun D *et al.* (2004). Impact of short-term haemodialysis catheters of the central veins: a catheter venographic study. *European Journal of Radiology* 52:293–299.

Oquzkurt L, Tercan F, Torun D *et al.* (2005). Ultrasound-guided placement of temporary IJV catheters: immediate technical success and complications in normal and high-risk patients. *European Journal of Radiology* 55:125–129.

Raad II *et al.* (1994). The relationship between the thrombotic and infectious complications of central venous catheters. *JAMA* 271:1014–1016.

Randolph AG, Cook DJ, Gonzales CA *et al.* (1996). Ultrasound guidance for placement of central venous catheters: a meta-analysis of the literature. *Critical Care Medicine* 24:2053–2058.

Reusch S, Walder B, Tramer MR *et al.* (2002). Complications of central venous catheters: internal jugular versus subclavian access – a systematic review. *Critical Care Medicine* 30:454–460.

Tercan F, Ozkan U, Oguzkurt L. *et al.* (2008). Ultrasound-guided placement of central venous catheters in patients with disorders of haemostasis. *European Journal of Radiology* 65:253–256.

Turba UC, Uflacker R, Hannegan *et al.* (2005). Anatomic relationship of internal jugular vein and common carotid artery applied to transjugular procedures. *Cardiovascular and Interventional Radiology* 28:303–306.

Wigmore TJ, Smythe JF, Hacking MB *et al.* (2007). Effect of the implementation of NICE guidelines for ultrasound guidance on the complication rates associated with central venous catheter placement in patients presenting for routine surgery in a tertiary referral centre. *British Journal of Anaesthesia* 99:662–665.

Chapter 6

Venous access via the femoral vein

Andrew Gratrix and Andrew R. Bodenham

Introduction

The femoral vein is widely used for central venous catheterisation. The technique of introducing a catheter into the inferior vena cava through a percutaneous puncture of the femoral vein was introduced by Duffy in 1949. It is often considered a safer option compared to other sites, but the anatomy is more complicated than commonly realised.

Anatomy of the femoral vein

The common femoral vein drains the majority of the blood from the lower limb as shown in Figure 6.1. It is usually cannulated at a level just below the inguinal ligament where the vessels lie in the configuration demonstrated in Figure 6.2. This area is at the base of the so-called femoral triangle which is a depressed area in the medial aspect of the thigh just below the inguinal ligament. Its superior border is the inguinal ligament, lateral border is the sartorius muscle, medial border is the adductor longus muscle and the floor is formed by the iliopsoas, pectineus and adductor longus muscles. The roof is formed by the skin and fasciae of the thigh. Other structures of note in the femoral triangle include the femoral nerve, the long saphenous vein and lymph nodes.

The femoral vein enters the thigh as a continuation of the popliteal vein. It ascends through the thigh, lying at first on the lateral side of the artery, then posterior to it and finally on its medial side. It leaves the thigh as it passes behind the inguinal ligament to become the external iliac vein. It should be appreciated that the overlap of the superficial femoral artery (SFA) over the femoral vein occurs much higher towards the inguinal ligament than is commonly realised, and anatomical drawings tend to omit this important anatomical relationship. The point of maximal pulsation in the groin will often be over the SFA rather than the common femoral artery. Using the point of maximal arterial pulsation as an anatomical landmark will often lead to the intended

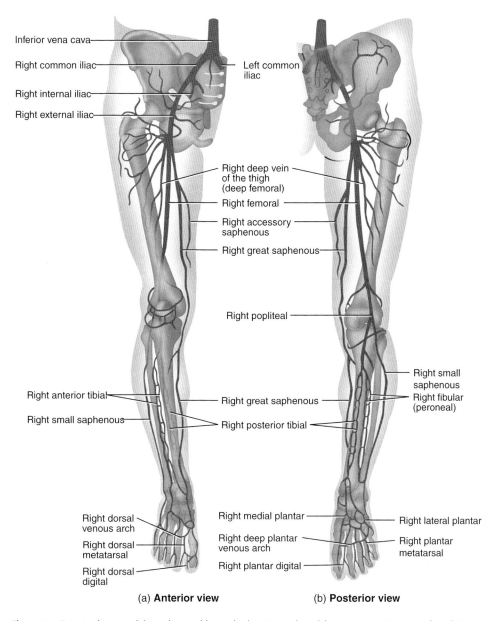

Inferior vena cava

Right common iliac

Right internal iliac

Right external iliac

Left common iliac

Right deep vein of the thigh (deep femoral)

Right femoral

Right accessory saphenous

Right great saphenous

Right popliteal

Right small saphenous

Right fibular (peroneal)

Right anterior tibial

Right great saphenous

Right small saphenous

Right posterior tibial

Right dorsal venous arch

Right medial plantar

Right lateral plantar

Right dorsal metatarsal

Right deep plantar venous arch

Right plantar metatarsal

Right dorsal digital

Right plantar digital

(a) Anterior view

(b) Posterior view

Figure 6.1 Principal veins of the pelvis and lower limbs. (Reproduced from Tortora GJ, *Principles of Human Anatomy*.)

puncture site for the femoral vein being too low with the vein in a relatively inaccessible position behind the artery. Similar problems ensue when cannulating the femoral artery. Often the SFA is entered, rather than the common femoral artery. Many punctures will be too low as skin creases do not indicate levels accurately and the inguinal ligament cannot be felt in the average subject.

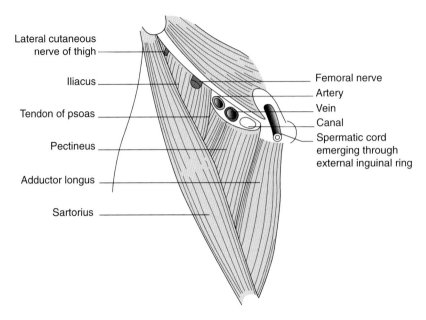

Figure 6.2 Anatomy of the femoral vessels at the level of the inguinal ligament. (Reproduced from Ellis H, *Clinical Anatomy* 2004, Figure 174, p. 238.)

Use of the femoral vein

This can be for either short- or long-term use. Advantages of the femoral approach include the straight route of access to the inferior vena cava (IVC) and its ease of access. As a result of its straight course, the long length of the IVC and the absence of the pleura, X-ray verification of the position of the catheter is not generally required. Relative contraindications to the use of this route include previous iliofemoral DVT, peripheral vascular disease, previous vascular surgery at this site (particularly if prosthetic graft is present), coagulopathy, infection or other dermatological conditions in the intertriginous fold. Documented thrombus in the vein or the presence of an IVC filter are absolute contraindications. Femoral catheters are uncomfortable and prone to dislodgement in the mobile patient.

Vascular access devices for the femoral approach

A large number of different devices can be used for femoral access ranging from standard single or multi-lumen central venous catheters and renal replacement catheters to larger bore catheters for cardiopulmonary bypass. Its straight course on both sides makes it a route of choice for larger bore stiffer catheters. All catheters are suitable for this route of access but length is important due to the mobility of the site and the distance to the IVC and right heart if access to this site is required. Short catheters will displace more easily with leg flexion. The femoral vein is widely used for interventional radiology and right heart catheterisation in adults and children.

Landmark technique

This was first described by Hohn and Lambert in 1966. Place the patient in a supine position and abduct and externally rotate the thigh. In a hypovolaemic patient, the vein may be filled by head-up tilt, or a Valsalva manoeuvre. Clean and prepare the skin and use local anaesthetic if indicated. Stand on the same side as the puncture site. Identify the femoral artery below the inguinal ligament (line from anterior iliac spine to pubic tubercle) by palpation. The vein is medial to the artery. Care is required to avoid puncture of the artery. Insert the needle 1–2 cm medial to the artery just below the inguinal ligament. Aim the needle cephalad. The vein is usually entered at about 2–4 cm deep. Once the vein is entered, advance the guidewire into the vein and remove the needle. A small incision is usually required to allow passage of the dilator. Pass the dilator into the vein using gentle pressure. Bear in mind that the catheter has to pass at a steep angle down into the vein and then its path flattens.

With deeper vessels in the larger patient, it may be difficult to pass large stiff dilators around the acute angle into the vein and a flatter puncture angle may sometimes be required. Remove the dilator and pass the catheter into the vein to the required length and remove the guidewire. Secure the catheter in position. If the artery is punctured inadvertently by the needle only, withdraw and apply firm timed pressure for at least 10 minutes. If larger dilators or catheters are inserted, leave in situ and seek senior advice, as there are closure devices available to seal arterial punctures or the device can be removed surgically and the artery sutured.

X-ray verification is not usually used but may be useful for longer-term access to ensure that there is no kinking and that catheter tip has not entered lumbar or other branches.

Use of ultrasound

This was reported by Sato *et al.* in 1998. The femoral vein may be scanned in transverse or longitudinal section. Care is needed to obtain correct orientation and correctly recognise the various vessels present. It is not easy to scan anteriorly above the inguinal ligament due to gas-filled loops of bowel in the peritoneal space. At the level of the inguinal ligament, the nerve, artery and vein lie in the characteristic cross-sectional orientation (Figure 6.3).

On descending from the inguinal ligament, the artery divides into the profunda and superficial femoral artery. The femoral vein receives a large tributary in the form of the long saphenous vein. Depending on exact orientation and anatomical level, these vessels may appear as a three or four leaf clover on ultrasound image. This is the so-called 'Mickey Mouse sign' (Figures 6.4a and 6.4b). Direct pressure through the probe enables the operator to distinguish arteries from veins.

Further verification of the vessel anatomy may be achieved using Doppler. Compression of the lower limb calf or thigh muscles will produce a venous pressure wave that can be seen by Doppler. In a conscious patient, the same effect is achieved by asking the patient to contract calf muscles. The vein should vary in size with respiration and a Valsalva manoeuvre. Intravascular thrombus can be seen with ultrasound scanning and further identified by the inability to compress and empty the vein completely. There

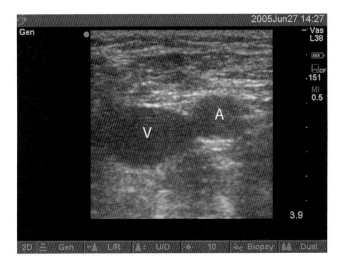

Figure 6.3 Ultrasound image of the left femoral artery and vein in cross section (as seen as if standing at the feet) immediately below the inguinal ligament. Depth of ultrasound image is 3.9 cm. A, artery; V, vein.

have been reports of distal femoral vein puncture below the femoral triangle using ultrasound to visualise the vein (Shang 2000), but to date there are no comparative trials comparing this to the traditional approaches higher up.

Technical considerations

Sterile precautions should be taken at all times. Preparation of equipment and patient should be undertaken including infiltration of local anaesthetic solution if being used. An assistant may be required to retract the abdominal wall in obese patients.

It is useful to perform a preliminary non-sterile scan to assess the vein for patency, size and thrombus. Put the ultrasound screen on the opposite side of the patient to where you are standing. The size of the veins will be enhanced by head-up tilt, a Valsalva manoeuvre or raising the patient's head. The right-hand side will be easier to access for a right-handed operator and vice versa. There is no documented anatomical advantage to one side or the other.

Following identification of the common femoral vein using ultrasound, insert the introducing needle either in transverse or longitudinal view until the needle tip is seen to indent and penetrate the anterior vein wall. The guidewire is then passed centrally, and its position travelling towards the abdomen can be visualised. The procedure is then completed in the usual way.

Temporary use of the femoral vein

The femoral vein can be used for temporary vascular access in situations such as intensive care patients, paediatrics, patients undergoing surgery, angiography, right heart

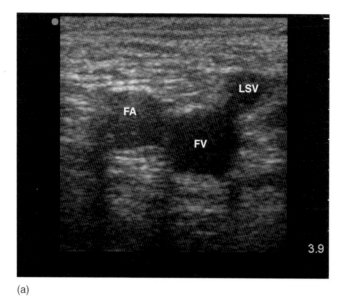

(a)

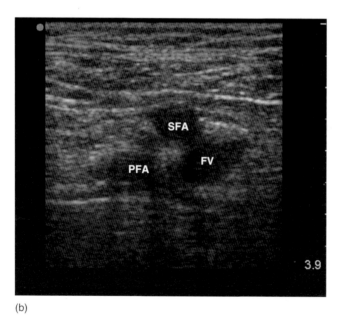

(b)

Figure 6.4 (a) Ultrasound image showing the 'Mickey Mouse sign' on left side (as seen if standing at feet), approximately 2 cm below the inguinal ligament. LSV, long saphenous vein draining into femoral vein (FV); FA, femoral artery. (b) Ultrasound image approximately 4 cm below the inguinal ligament where the femoral artery divides into superficial (SFA) and deep (profunda femoris, PFA) branches. The SFA partially overlaps the FV. Depth of ultrasound image is 3.9 cm.

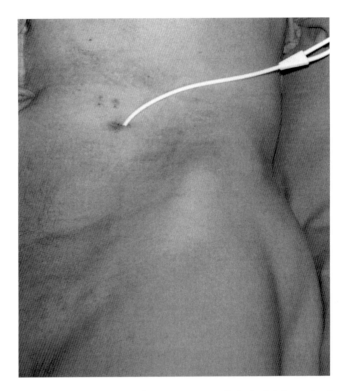

Figure 6.5 Hickman line in patient with SVC obstruction, inserted via the left femoral vein and tunnelled upwards to umbilical level on the abdominal wall. The puncture site in the groin is healed.

catheters and temporary pacemakers. It is also useful for large stiff catheters such as renal dialysis catheters and cardiopulmonary bypass catheters.

Long-term use of the femoral vein

The femoral vein can be used for long-term vascular access (Kaufman 2002) in situations where the other accessible veins are unable to be used, e.g. superior vena cava obstruction. The line is tunnelled onto the abdominal wall or thigh to move the access site away from the skin folds (Figure 6.5).

Catheter tip position

There is no consensus as to the optimum site of catheter tip, which dependening on length and the size of the patient will lie somewhere between iliac vessels, low IVC, the intrahepatic IVC, or right atrium. Most standard length catheters (20 cm) are only likely to reach the iliac veins or lower IVC. The right atrium will be approximately 30–40 cm away from the common femoral vein in an adult male. For dialysis catheters, ensure that the tip is within the IVC to avoid recirculation of blood, i.e. use a 25-cm catheter. For long-term catheters, it may be useful to check for position, kinking and flow by X-ray fluoroscopy, contrast or ultrasound to confirm good tip position.

Advantages and disadvantages of femoral venous access

Advantages of the femoral approach are discussed above.

Operators should be aware of complications of femoral venous access. Haemorrhage from the femoral artery may result in haematoma or false aneurysm requiring compression or surgical exploration (Figure 6.6). The proximity of the arteries and vein allow the potential development of AV fistulae if both vessels are punctured simultaneously. It should also be noted that blood can track upwards into the retroperitoneal and then into the peritoneal space causing possible concealed fatal haemorrhage. Damage can also occur to nerves and lymphatics in the area. If the catheter is misplaced or inserted to insufficient depth, extravasation of the infused solution can occur. Other complications include thrombophlebitis, thrombosis, catheter-related infection and sepsis.

Merrer *et al.*(2001) showed that the infection rate (19.8% versus 4.5%) and thrombosis rate (21.5% versus 1.9%) are higher when using the femoral vein compared to the subclavian vein. Other studies have not shown this difference (Stenzel *et al.* 1989, Montagnac *et al.* 1997, Still *et al.* 1998, Deshpande *et al.* 2005). It is speculated that differences in infection and thrombosis rates may be due to the close approximation to urine and faeces and the less clean nature of the site. The femoral vein is often the last vein to be used in rotation in patients with high risks of sepsis and thrombosis when other sites are exhausted. It is also often the first choice in emergency conditions because of ease of access, but here strict sterile conditions may be overlooked. Such

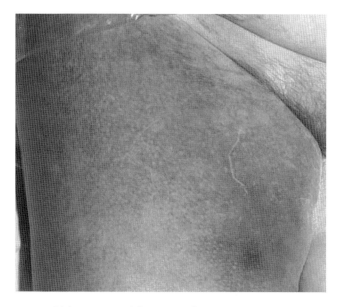

Figure 6.6 Haematoma and false aneurysm following inadvertent arterial puncture during attempted blind landmark puncture of right femoral vein for a dialysis catheter on ICU.

considerations dictate that the choice of access site should be individualised for each patient dependent on their characteristics and choice, plus the competence of the operator at each site.

The femoral vein is ideal for short-term access in catheter lab, theatres, etc., but less so for longer-term use in ICU or true long-term access but clinical compromises are required and each decision made on an individual basis.

Removal

Vascular devices may be removed from the femoral vein with comparative ease. Always ensure sterile technique. Remove sutures and/or dressings. Remove catheter by gentle traction and press on puncture site with sterile gauze until bleeding stops. Dress the site with sterile dressing.

Conclusion

The femoral vein can be used for all forms of vascular access both short and long term, using a variety of techniques. This route is both safe and practical for a variety of procedures and should not be automatically overlooked in favour of other routes. The relative risk on benefits compared to other sites should be individually considered for each patient.

References

Deshpande KS, Hatem C, Ulrich HL *et al.* (2005). The incidence of infectious complications of central venous catheters at the subclavian, internal jugular, and femoral sites in an intensive care unit population. *Critical Care Medicine* 33:13–20.

Duffy BJ (1949). The clinical use of polyethylene tubing for intravenous therapy. *Annals of Surgery* 130:929.

Hohn AR, Lambert EC (1966). Continuous venous catheterisation in children. *JAMA* 197:658.

Kaufman JA (2002). Alternative routes of catheter placement. In *Venous Catheters: A Practical Manual*, Pieters PC, Tisnado J, Mauro MA *et al.* (eds), Thieme, New York, pp. 190–207.

Merrer J, De Jonghe B, Golliot F *et al.* (2001). Complications of femoral and subclavian venous catheterisation in critically ill patients. *JAMA* 286:700–707.

Montagnac R, Bernard C, Guillaumie J *et al.* (1997). Indwelling silicone femoral catheters: experience of three haemodialysis centres. *Nephrology, Dialysis, Transplantation* 12:772–775.

Sato S, Ueno E, Toyooka H (1998). Central venous access via the distal femoral vein using ultrasound guidance. *Anaesthesiology* 88:838.

Shang NG (2000). The femoral vein. In *Percutaneous Central Venous and Arterial Catheterisation*, Latto IP, Jones PL, Nq WS *et al.* (ed.), WB Saunders, London, UK, pp. 211–221.

Stenzel JP, Green TP, Fuhrman BP *et al.* (1989). Percutaneous femoral venous catheterisations: a prospective study of complications. *Journal of Pediatrics* 114:411–415.

Still JM, Law E, Thiruvaiyaru D *et al.* (1998). Central line-related sepsis in acute burn patients. *American Surgeon* 64:165–170.

Chapter 7

Central venous access via the subclavian and axillary veins

Simon Galloway and Andrew R. Bodenham

Introduction

The axillary–subclavian vein complex has been a standard route of access to the central venous circulation. First described in 1952 by Aubaniac, the subclavian route of venous access resolved many of the problems associated with the well-established external jugular route, most notably failure to pass the catheter centrally. Axillary vein cannulation was first described by Spracklen *et al.* (1967) via an axillary route as an attempt to reduce the inherent risk of pneumothorax associated with the subclavian route. This was followed by an alternative infraclavicular technique (Nickalls 1987). The use of ultrasound to aid in examination of the anatomy (Galloway and Bodenham 2003) and subsequently with cannulation has improved the safety and accuracy of the axillary/subclavian route (Sandhu 2004, Sharma *et al.* 2004).

The supraclavicular approach to the subclavian vein, first suggested by Yoffa in 1965, has its advocates but has never gained widespread popularity. Both veins and all routes have been used for a wide range of therapeutic and diagnostic indications.

This chapter describes the applied venous anatomy and the indications and contraindications to each route. Each route is described and the advantages and disadvantages are discussed.

Applied anatomy

The axillary vein is the continuation of the basilic vein and extends from the outer border of the teres major muscle to the outer border of the first rib. The vein runs upwards on the medial side of the axillary artery to this point where it continues as the

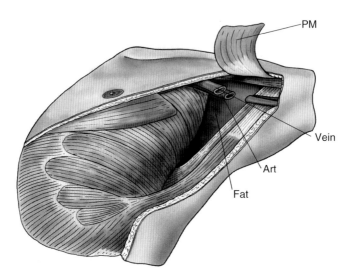

Figure 7.1 Anatomy of the infraclavicular region. The pectoralis minor muscle has been reflected to facilitate the view. Note the area lateral to the rib cage. This contains only axillary fat. Vein, axillary vein; Art, axillary artery; PM, pectoralis minor muscle; Fat, axillary fat. (Reprinted from Galloway and Bodenham 2003, with permission from *British Journal of Anaesthesia*.)

subclavian vein. Its route from deep in the axilla takes it on a course that runs from lateral to medial, inferior to superior and posterior to anterior (Figure 7.1).

The axillary vein is crossed immediately anteriorly by the pectoralis minor muscle, which divides the vein topographically into three parts, namely proximal, posterior and distal (these names are with regard to the pectoralis minor muscle). The axillary vein receives the cephalic vein from above. As it passes more medially, the axillary vein becomes larger, more superficial and more closely applied to the axillary artery. In addition, the vein and pleura are more closely related at the medial end. This means that there is a compromise when attempting to access the axillary vein. A medial axillary cannulation provides a larger, more superficial vessel allowing easier cannulation, but the proximity of the axillary artery and pleura increase the risk of complication. This dilemma is easily resolved with the use of ultrasound to allow visualization of the most beneficial site and to avoid unwanted puncture of neighbouring structures (Figures 7.2 and 7.3).

The subclavian vein is a continuation of the axillary vein from the outer border of the first rib to the medial border of the scalenus anterior muscle. Here it joins the internal jugular vein to form the brachiocephalic vein behind the sternoclavicular joint (Figure 7.4).

On the left, the subclavian vein receives the valved termination of the thoracic duct. The lymph from the major part of the body drains into the thoracic duct from the regional lymph nodes. Lymph from the right upper quadrant drains into the right lymphatic duct which joins the right subclavian vein at its junction with the right internal jugular vein (Figure 7.4). The right lymphatic duct is much smaller than the thoracic duct and so is less likely to be damaged or give rise to symptoms of damage. The thoracic duct is potentially damaged during a left-sided subclavian vein puncture and if

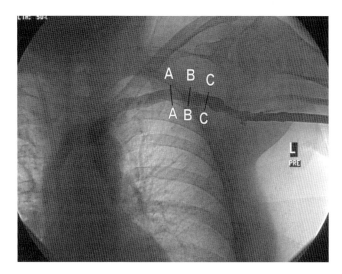

Figure 7.2 Appearance of a normal left axillary venogram. Contrast has been injected into a peripheral vein. Note the irregular outline of the vein due to venous valves. Some contrast is also seen in the cephalic vein. The axillary vein is seen draining into the brachiocephalic system. The line A–A represents the scan for Figure 7.3a. The line B–B represents the scan for Figure 7.3b. The line C–C represents the scan for Figure 7.3c. (Reprinted from Galloway and Bodenham 2003, with permission from *British Journal of Anaesthesia*.)

lymph leaks into the pleural space a so-called 'chylothorax' forms. Chyle (clear lymph fluid from tissues, plus oily chylomicrons from the gut) is oily white in appearance if the patient is being fed enterally. In addition, thrombosis of the left subclavian vein (a recognised complication of venous access) can cause a blockage in lymphatic drainage (Mallick and Bodenham 2003).

The close relationship between the axillary vein and the apex of the lung is continued when it becomes the subclavian vein. The subclavian vein is difficult to visualise with ultrasound. In some individuals, the vein is in the form of a plexus, in such cases cannulation should not be attempted and access should be sought at another site.

Thrombus in the axillary vein is usually evident clinically by the presence of arm swelling and is easily seen on ultrasound. This contrasts with thrombus in the internal jugular vein which is usually silent if unilateral.

The limited space where the subclavian vein passes between the clavicle and first rib can cause a condition known as 'pinch-off'. A triangle is formed by the clavicle, first rib and costoclavicular ligament. Catheters passing extravascularly through this space can be compressed, leading to catheter blockage or rupture (Figures 7.5a–7.5c). Catheters inserted more laterally will pass through this space intravascularly and should be less likely to be compressed (Aitken and Minton 1984). A high index of suspicion is required and catheters which only flush or aspirate with the arm abducted or show compression on X-ray should be assumed to be pinching off. Removal should be considered as soon as possible before fracture occurs (De Graaff *et al.* 2006).

The artery runs a parallel course to the vein and underlies it more medially, making it vulnerable in landmark subclavian techniques even if the needle alignment is correct to the vein. Medial to the first rib it indents the pleural space covered only by pleura; damage to the artery at this site may lead to massive bleeding into the low-pressure

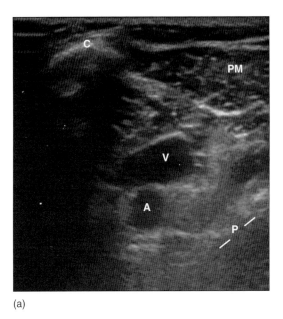

(a)

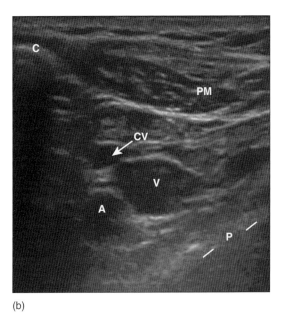

(b)

Figure 7.3 Ultrasound anatomy of the right axillary vein as viewed from the right, depth of image 4 cm. C: clavicle; V: axillary vein; A: axillary artery; P: chest wall/pleura; CV: cephalic vein; PM: pectoralis minor. Note the anatomical changes on moving from medial to lateral (a)–(b)–(c). The overlap of vein and artery reduces.

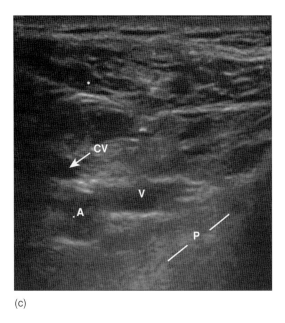

(c)

Figure 7.3 (*Continued*)

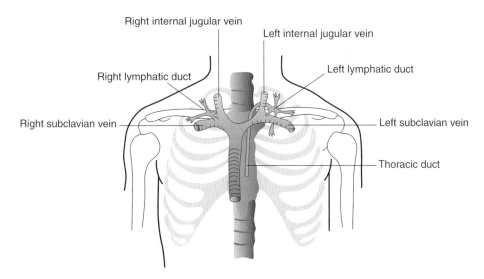

Figure 7.4 Anatomy of the subclavian vein, axillary vein and thoracic duct. The subclavian vein is a continuation of the axillary vein. It joins the internal jugular vein to form the brachiocephalic vein behind the sternoclavicular joint. On the left, the subclavian vein receives the valved termination of the thoracic duct. The lymph from the major part of the body drains into the thoracic duct from the regional lymph nodes. Lymph from the right upper quadrant drains into the right lymphatic duct.

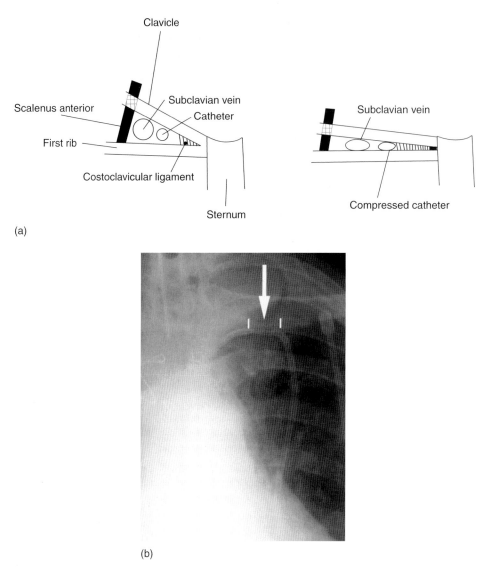

(a)

(b)

Figure 7.5 Pinch-off. (a) Mechanism of pinch-off. At catheter insertion, there is a wide angle between clavicle and first rib (left). This closes in the upright position (right). Catheters are at risk of compression. (Redrawn from Aitken and Minton 1984.) (b) Close-up view of left upper portion of chest X-ray. A single lumen Hickman catheter has been inserted via the left subclavian route. The section of catheter lying under the first rib and clavicle (arrow) shows characteristic compression (scalloping) suggestive of pinch-off. This catheter is at risk of rupture. (Reprinted from Galloway and Bodenham 2004, with permission from *British Journal of Anaesthesia.*) (c) Hickman catheter following rupture secondary to pinch-off. Note extravasation of radiological contrast (C).

pleural space. Small arterial branches can be seen with ultrasound crossing the vein and should be avoided. In thin patients, the artery can be palpated in this area. The brachial plexus lies closely in relation to the artery rather than the vein hence should be avoidable with ultrasound needle guidance towards the vein. This relationship has been well investigated in magnetic resonance imaging-based studies (Wilson *et al.* 1998).

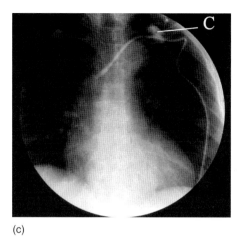

(c)

Figure 7.5 *(Continued)*

Insertion techniques

Sterile precautions should be taken for all central venous cannulation procedures. Preparation of equipment and infiltration of local anaesthetic should be carried out using aseptic technique and the presence of an assistant is beneficial. Any standard Seldinger technique central venous catheter can be used, but large stiff catheters may be difficult to traverse round corners into the superior vena cava (SVC) (such angulation may be much more marked than anatomical texts suggest).

Landmark infraclavicular subclavian vein puncture

Position the patient supine and slightly head down. This distends the vein and reduces the risk of air embolus. Many approaches have been described (Latto 1992) but none is ideal. A finger is inserted in the subclavian groove and pressed medially until resistance is felt. This corresponds to the subclavius muscle. The needle is inserted below the clavicle at this point, which will be at the junction of the medial and middle thirds of the clavicle (Figure 7.6a). The needle is passed towards the sternoclavicular joint and suprasternal notch (Figure 7.6b). Aspiration with the syringe during passage of the needle ensures that puncture of the vein is recognised. The vein is often transfixed with the needle. Thus, it is important to continue aspiration on withdrawal of the needle. A wire is passed through the needle and thereafter a standard Seldinger technique is used. It must be remembered that the stiff dilators need only be passed into the vein and not pushed 'to the hilt'. Noting the length of needle inserted prior to vein puncture will allow determination of required depth of dilator insertion. Excessive depth of dilator insertion can lead to vein trauma, causing thrombosis or potentially rupture.

Landmark-based techniques are inevitably compromised by anatomical variability. Variability in the anatomy of the subclavian vein is well described (Borja and Hinshaw 1970). This disadvantage combined with the proximity of the subclavian artery, brachial plexus and apical pleura leads to the well-recognised complications of pneumothorax

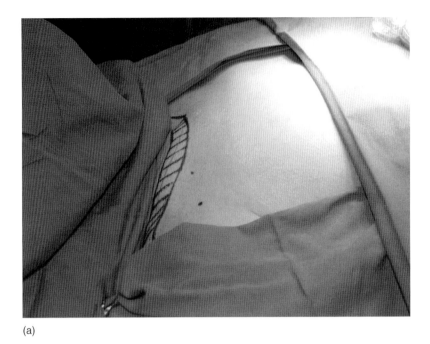

(a)

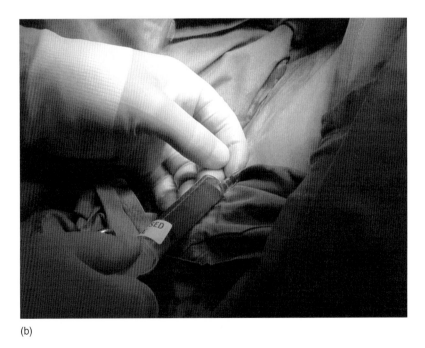

(b)

Figure 7.6 (a) Landmarks for right infraclavicular subclavian vein puncture. Puncture below clavicle (shaded) is usually at the junction of medial and middle thirds (medial dot). Ultrasound guided axillary vein puncture uses more lateral approach (lateral dot), although the exact location varies according to the ultrasound view. (b) Subclavian vein puncture. Note shallow angle of approach.

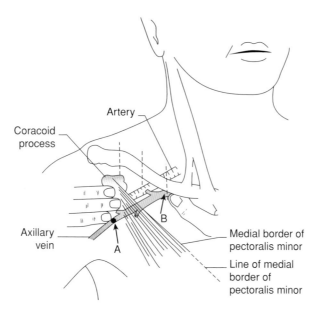

Figure 7.7 Landmark-based infraclavicular axillary vein puncture. Puncture site is three fingerbreadths below the coracoid process. The needle is aimed towards the medial end of the clavicle. (Reprinted from Nickalls 1987, with permission from Blackwell Publishing.)

and arterial puncture and the less common neuropraxia. The position of the subclavian artery causes further difficulty if it is accidentally punctured as it cannot be easily compressed to reduce haematoma formation. A further disadvantage, particularly compared to the internal jugular route, is the curved route of insertion. This can cause a failure to achieve central positioning due to guide wire misdirection. There is, however, greater patient comfort (Untracht 1988) and easier fixation for catheters inserted via the subclavian vein. In addition, there is a perceived reduction in sepsis and thrombosis compared to other routes (Stenzel *et al.* 1989, Montagnac *et al.* 1997, Still *et al.* 1998, Merrer *et al.* 2001, Deshpande *et al.* 2005). Thrombosis is more obvious than in the internal jugular vein as described above.

Central passage of catheters can be helped by turning the patients head away and applying pressure on the internal jugular vein to close it. In addition, in awake patients, a deep inspiration may aid central passage.

Axillary vein

Landmark-based infraclavicular axillary vein puncture has been described using an insertion point three fingerbreadths below the coracoid process slightly lateral to the lateral border of pectoralis minor. The needle is aimed towards the point just below the medial end of the clavicle (Figure 7.7) (Nickalls 1987). This technique never gained widespread acceptance and has been largely superseded by ultrasound-guided techniques.

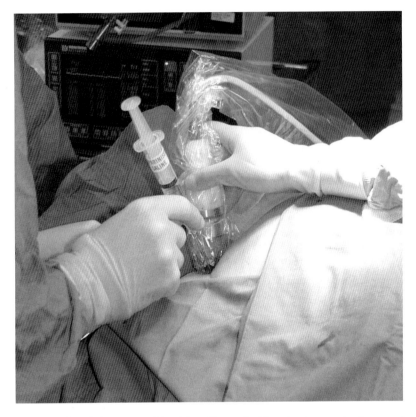

Figure 7.8 Ultrasound guided puncture of the right axillary vein. Note the steep angle of approach.

Ultrasound-guided axillary vein cannulation

Using an ultrasound device with a 5–10 MHz probe, the vessels are imaged in cross section together with the chest wall medially. The vessels appear as non-echogenic circular structures. The artery is pulsatile and non-compressible and is seen more easily with probe compression. The vein is non-pulsatile (but may have transmitted movements from the adjacent artery) and can be compressed with pressure from the ultrasound probe. The cephalic vein can be seen as a major tributary of the axillary vein. There is marked respiratory variation in vein size in the spontaneously breathing patient particularly if they are hypovolaemic. The needle is advanced at a steep angle towards the vein, guided by the ultrasound probe orientation (Figure 7.8, see also Chapter 9) either in short or long axis. The needle tip can be visualised either as a bright spot or by local tissue distortion. Needle advancement with constant aspiration allows confirmation of the vein puncture. Passage of a wire through the needle allows a normal Seldinger technique to be used. Although straighter than the subclavian vein, similar precautions should be taken in terms of passage of stiff dilators.

The axillary vein has all of the advantages associated with the subclavian vein in terms of comfort, ease of fixation and risk of infection. In addition, there is a reduced risk of pinch-off and in the event of accidental arterial puncture the vessels are easily compressible. Inadvertent arterial puncture can be repaired by surgical cut down without clavicle resection. This approach is identical to that taken in an axillo-femoral bypass dissection. Haematoma from the axillary artery spreads laterally to the upper arm rather than into the chest. The use of ultrasound-guided techniques allows selection of the most favourable site. It allows the practitioner to select a section of patent vein that is not closely applied to the artery or pleura. This will reduce the complication rate and failure rate of venous cannulation. Arterial and pleural puncture should be virtually eliminated. Puncture with ultrasound guidance via the axilla can be used but is not a clean dry site and cannot be recommended except for short-term use.

Supraclavicular

The subclavian vein can be accessed via a supraclavicular route, but this route has never been as popular as the infraclavicular route. This route involves inserting a needle through a point joining the medial and middle thirds of the clavicle and about 2 cm above it. This point corresponds to the lateral border of the clavicular head of the sternocleidomastoid muscle. The needle is inserted medially and caudally towards the subclavian vein about 2–3 cm behind the sternoclavicular joint. Ultrasound can be used to guide vein puncture. The vein and artery can be seen posterior to the clavicle over the first rib. The vein is partially covered by the clavicle. Puncture procedure is then similar to other sites. A significant advantage of the right supraclavicular puncture is that the superior puncture site in the vein is in a medial position adjacent to the confluence of subclavian and internal jugular veins. This means that catheters run a nearly straight course to the SVC. This means blind central placement is more likely and stiffer larger catheters and dilators do not have to round a corner. The left side is less favourable in this respect. An interesting approach has been described in the smaller child where the supraclavicular section of the vein is visualised in longitudinal section with ultrasound whilst the introducing needle is introduced under the clavicle into the vein (Pirotte and Veyckemans 2007).

Use of the subclavian and axillary veins

The subclavian and axillary veins can be used for almost all short- and long-term indications. They are commonly used for long-term access with Hickman-type catheters and ports. In addition, they are often the veins of choice for cardiac pacing and long-term total parenteral nutrition. However, the curved route of access makes it more difficult to use very stiff catheters and they increase the risk of vessel wall damage. It should be noted that renal failure patients who will require dialysis need patent veins for arterio-venous fistula formation, so these veins should be avoided. In addition, venous pressures are higher in the presence of an existing arterio-venous fistula. As a result, there is a markedly increased bleeding risk. The site is also relatively contraindicated in the patient who has had an axillary node clearance for breast carcinoma with secondary lymphoedema in whom thrombosis may be a major problem in an already compromised limb.

Tip position with central venous catheters inserted via the axillary or subclavian veins is critical. The tip should ideally lie within the SVC, in the long axis of the vein. The tip should not be abutting the vein wall at an acute angle. It has been recommended that the catheter tip should lie above the pericardial reflection (Fletcher and Bodenham 2000, Stonelake and Bodenham 2006). This is to avoid the risk of perforation and tamponade that can occur if the catheter tip is within the heart. The carina can be used to define the upper limit of the pericardium on a post-procedure chest X-ray. It is also noteworthy that the catheter tip will move between lying and sitting positions. It may not be possible to achieve adequate tip position and direction in the SVC with left-sided catheters without allowing them to lie below the carina. This may mean that the tip lies within the right atrium.

Conclusion

The axillary and subclavian veins provide comfortable, acceptable sites for central venous access with a low risk of infection. The subclavian vein has long been a mainstay of medical practice, despite the risk of pneumothorax. The axillary vein, despite lower popularity, provides a useful alternative site for venous access, particularly when accessed with ultrasound guidance.

References

Aitken D, Minton J (1984). The 'pinch-off sign': a warning of impending problems with permanent subclavian catheters. *American Journal of Surgery* 148:633–636.

Aubaniac R (1952). L'injection intraveineuse sous-claviculaire. *Presse Medicale* 60:1456.

Borja AR, Hinshaw JR (1970). A safe way to perform infraclavicular subclavian vein catheterization. *Surgery, Gynecology & Obstetrics* 130:673–676.

De Graaff J, Bras L, Vos J (2006). Early transection of a central venous catheter in a sedated ICU patient. *British Journal of Anaesthesia* 97:832–834.

Deshpande KS, Hatem C, Ulrich HL *et al.* (2005). The incidence of infectious complications of central venous catheters at the subclavian, internal jugular, and femoral sites in an intensive care unit population. *Critical Care Medicine* 33:13–20.

Fletcher S, Bodenham A (2000). Safe placement of central venous catheters: where should the tip of the catheter lie? *British Journal of Anaesthesia* 85:188–191.

Galloway S, Bodenham A (2003). Ultrasound imaging of the axillary vein – anatomical basis for central venous access. *British Journal of Anaesthesia* 5:589–595.

Galloway S, Bodenham A (2004). Long-term central venous access. *British Journal of Anaesthesia* 92:722–734.

Latto IP (1992). The subclavian vein. In *Percutaneous Central Venous and Arterial Catheterisation*, Latto IP, Ng WS, Jones PL *et al.* (eds), Harcourt Publishers, London, UK, pp. 78–90.

Mallick A, Bodenham A (2003). Disorders of the lymph circulation: their relevance to anaesthesia and intensive care. *British Journal of Anaesthesia* 91:265–272.

Merrer J, De Jonghe B, Golliot F *et al.* (2001). Complications of femoral and subclavian venous catheterisation in critically ill patients. *JAMA* 286:700–707.

Montagnac R, Bernard C, Guillaumie J *et al.* (1997). Indwelling silicone femoral catheters: experience of three haemodialysis centres. *Nephrology, Dialysis, Transplantation* 12:772–775.

Nickalls RWD (1987). A new percutaneous infraclavicular approach to the axillary vein. *Anaesthesia* 42:151–154.

Pirotte T, Veyckemans F (2007). Ultrasound-guided subclavian vein cannulation in infants and children: a novel approach. *British Journal of Anaesthesia* 98:509–514.

Sandhu N (2004). Transpectoral ultrasound guided catheterization of the axillary vein: an alternative to standard catheterization of the subclavian vein. *Anesthesia and Analgesia* 99:183–187.

Sharma A, Bodenham A, Mallick A (2004). Ultrasound-guided infraclavicular axillary vein cannulation for central venous access. *British Journal of Anaesthesia* 93:188–192.

Spracklen F, Niesche F, Lord P *et al.* (1967). Percutaneous catheterization of the axillary vein. *Cardiovascular Research* 1:297–300.

Stenzel JP, Green TP, Fuhrman BP *et al.* (1989). Percutaneous femoral venous catheterisations: a prospective study of complications. *Journal of Pediatrics* 114:411–415.

Still JM, Law E, Thiruvaiyaru D *et al.* (1998). Central line-related sepsis in acute burn patients. *American Surgeon* 64:165–170.

Stonelake P, Bodenham A (2006). The carina as a radiological landmark for central venous catheter tip position. *British Journal of Anaesthesia* 96:335–340.

Untracht S (1988). Axillary artery as a landmark in cannulating the subclavian vein. *Surgery, Gynecology & Obstetrics* 166:565–566.

Wilson J, Brown D, Wong G *et al.* (1998). Infraclavicular brachial plexus block: parasagittal anatomy important to the coracoid technique. *Anesthesia and Analgesia* 87:870–873.

Yoffa D (1965). Supraclavicular subclavian venepuncture and catheterisation. *Lancet* 2:614–617.

Chapter 8

Peripherally inserted central catheters

Nancy Moureau and Janice Gabriel

Introduction

Early selection of the most appropriate IV catheter will result in safer, more efficient administration of IV therapy, leading to greater patient satisfaction, reduced overall nursing time for IV maintenance, cost savings, fewer supplies, reduced risk of complications and a greater chance of the patient completing their prescribed treatment (Moreau *et al.* 2002). The first thought is often to start with a peripheral intravenous device which is the most widely used and least expensive device available, although is not always the most appropriate choice for an individual patient and their prescribed therapy. Careful considerations for the length of therapy, medication characteristics, diagnosis and, where appropriate, patient preference should all be assessed to determine the most appropriate choice for each individual patient.

Objectives

- Comparison of the patient selection criteria and clinical indications for the use of a PICC compared to a midline or peripheral device.
- Identification of indications, contraindications and benefits associated with peripherally inserted central catheters (PICCs).
- Understanding the differences between the over the needle peel-away insertion of a PICC compared to modified Seldinger techniques (MST).
- Evaluation of the benefits of ultrasound guided PICC insertion.

Peripherally inserted central catheters

PICCs are a group of single, dual and triple lumen central venous access devices (CVADs), which were developed in the late 1970s in the USA (Gabriel 1996a, Dougherty 2006, Nakazawa 2006). PICC gauge sizes vary from 15 to 28 gauges/1–7 Fr. They are available as open-ended catheters or with valves which can be incorporated into either the distal or proximal end of the device. These valves are designed so that in the absence of a negative or positive pressure they remain closed and thereby minimise the potential for reflux of blood (see Chapter 4) (Gabriel 2006). This chapter is largely concerned with devices designed for medium to long-term use, but there are also devices for short-term use that are used in anaesthesia and critical care. As PICCs are CVADs, they can be used for a range of infusions including vesicants (Dougherty 2006). Venous access is achieved by cannulating a peripheral vein in the arm, i.e. the cephalic, basilic or median cubital vein. The catheter is then advanced through the cannula, or introducer, until it reaches the superior vena cava (SVC) or right atrium (RA) (Figure 8.1).

As the diameter of the arm veins are smaller than the larger veins in the chest, too large a device for the vein could lead to mechanical phlebitis due to the irritation of the tunica intima by the catheter material. Therefore, triple lumen PICCs should be placed in either the cephalic or basilic vein higher up the patient's arm using a modified Seldinger technique (Gabriel 2008).

Originally, PICCs were designed for intermediate length parenteral therapies, i.e. not exceeding 12 weeks, but with good initial patient assessment and careful management they have been demonstrated to meet the clinical needs of patients for longer periods of time (Gabriel 2000).

As with any CVAD, radiology confirmation of tip position by either X-ray or fluoroscopy is required to verify SVC placement before using a PICC (RCN 2005, Dougherty 2006).

Midline catheters

Midline catheters are peripherally inserted catheters (PICs) with tip location not extending beyond the axillary vein (Figure 8.1). If a PICC intended for the SVC, falls short and terminates in the innominate/brachiocephalic vein, it should not be considered a central venous device and thus subject to the same limitations as a midline catheter (RCN 2005, Griffiths 2007).

Placement indications for midline catheters include:

- Hydrating intravenous fluids
- Short- to medium-term antibiotic administration with a non-irritating medication (pH 5–9, osmolarity less than 600 mOsm/L)
- Analgesia and sedation

Radiological confirmation is not necessary for midline catheter placement. Dwell time for these catheters is generally 2–6 weeks (RCN 2005, Griffiths 2007). Midline catheters are a suitable and more comfortable alternative to peripheral venous access for patients requiring short- to medium-term parenteral therapy. Management of a midline catheter is similar to a PICC (see below).

Patient assessment

Decision trees, algorithms, care pathways and other types of flow charts can be used to assist the vascular access device (VAD) selection process for an individual patient.

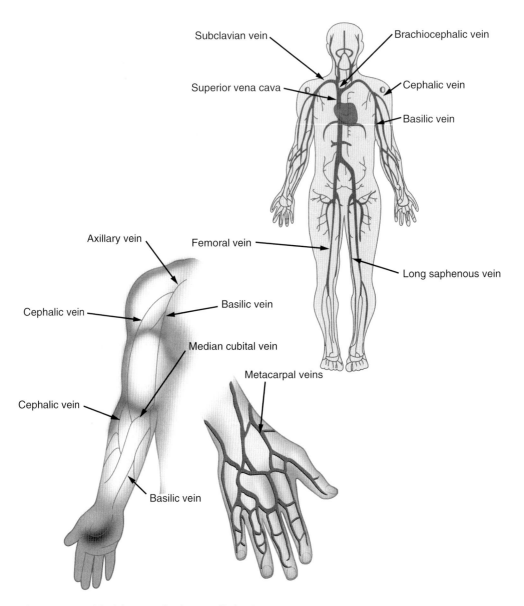

Figure 8.1 Simplified diagram of right upper limb veins.

Ideally, the most appropriate catheter is placed at the commencement of the patient's treatment, thereby allowing one device to be used for the entire length of their therapy. This is not only more comfortable for the patient, but careful patient assessment will result in less VAD-related complications and has the additional bonus of being cost-effective (Gabriel 2008).

Selection of patients

Before any VAD is placed it is crucial to undertake a thorough assessment of the individual patient (RCN 2005, Dougherty 2006, Gabriel 2006, Griffiths 2007) (see also Chapter 4).

Such an assessment should include:

- Underlying diagnosis, past history and age of patient
- Intended choice and duration of parenteral therapy
- Where the treatment will take place (e.g. inpatient, outpatient, home or self-administered)
- Condition of the limb and veins (if intending to place peripheral VAD)
- Previous problems with venepuncture and VADs
- Contraindications for placement site of CVAD
- Anaesthetic techniques
- Patient preference

Intended treatment/duration

When considering which device to place, thought needs to be given to the potential effects of the drugs/infusates on the patient's veins.

- Is the intended treatment vesicant or highly irritant to veins, e.g. sodium bicarbonate, vesicant cytotoxic drugs?
- Will large volumes of fluids require infusing, e.g. total parenteral nutrition (TPN)?
- Is the treatment intended to last for a few hours or continue over several weeks/months?

A peripheral cannula or midline catheter would probably suffice for treatment which lasted no more than a few days, and which is unlikely to cause problems for the patient's veins (pH neutral/low osmolarity). A CVAD would be a more appropriate device for a highly irritant treatment (alkaline/acidic or high osmolarity) and/or one likely to continue for several weeks/months (Dougherty 2006).

Location of treatment

Attention needs to be given to the intended location for treatment. If it is going to be wholly hospital based, then it is reasonable to assume there will be staff available who are knowledgeable and skilled to manage the patient's VAD. If the patient is to receive their treatment as an outpatient, or in the community, whatever device is placed, it must be a decision taken in conjunction with the patient, so they have the basic knowledge to care for their own device safely when away from the hospital environment. The degree of care required by the patient will vary on an individual basis, but as an absolute minimum it should include basic information about what the limitations of having such a device in situ may impose on them, and who to contact if they have a problem. Some patients may be totally self-caring of their own device, and administer their own parenteral therapies, such as a patient who has cystic fibrosis. These individuals will require the appropriate information, equipment, drugs and sharps boxes to manage their device safely (Kayley 2003). For the community nurse visiting patients requiring parenteral therapy, they must have ready access, together with sufficient supplies, of equipment and drugs, and unhindered access to safe disposal of used equipment (Kayley 2003).

Condition of limb and veins

If the patient has an oedematous arm, as a consequence of lymphoedema, trauma, an infected wound, dialysis shunt or other problems, then this limb should be avoided for cannulation, if at all possible, to reduce the potential for infection and discomfort for the patient (Hadaway 2006, Griffiths 2007).

It has been suggested that little attention is paid to veins, other than to view them as a means of obtaining venous access. As we age, the loss of connective tissue can result in fragile veins which can easily be damaged by the trauma of venepuncture, and make venepuncture/cannulation more challenging for both the patient and staff (Schelper 2003).

When assessing a patient for a peripheral VAD, it is advisable to site the device in the most suitable distal vein. This will provide the option of resiting a subsequent VAD above the first one, with a lower potential for infiltration/extravasation from leakage of the infusion/drug through an earlier venepuncture site. If re-siting of a VAD is required, ideally it should be placed in the opposite arm, but this is not always an option (RCN 2005, Dougherty 2008).

Previous problems with venepunctures/VADs

The placement of a PICC is usually a planned procedure, and the patient should be asked if they have experienced any previous problems with venepunctures or cannulation (Griffiths 2007, Gabriel 2008) (see Chapter 4). Careful planning can avoid most problems and increase the uneventful longevity of the PICC, and realise financial savings for the organisation by avoiding the need to place a new device or manage complications (Gabriel 2006).

Relevant medical history

Knowledge of the patient's medical history is crucial when assessing them for any VAD. If the patient has a bleeding tendency, it would be inappropriate to go ahead with the placement of a PICC without undertaking a blood count and coagulation screen. The placement of a PICC can be undertaken with care in patients with a bleeding tendency. Pressure can be applied to the PICC cannulation site until bleeding has stopped, **but this should be undertaken with care.** (Gabriel 1996b). The insertion site can also be easily observed for bleeding/haematoma formation. However, this should be discussed with the clinician in charge of their care before a decision is made to go ahead with the procedure (Dougherty 2006, Gabriel 2008).

Contraindications for placement sites of PICCs

If the patient is being considered for the placement of a PICC, the assessment should take into consideration the route of passage of the catheter from its insertion site to its ultimate termination in the SVC (Figure 8.1). Conditions which can impede the passage of the catheter through the vein can include:

- Enlarged axillary/supraclavicular lymph nodes
- Previous surgery/radiotherapy to the axilla/supraclavicular fossa
- Tumour mass
- Previous history of thrombosis
- History of fractured clavicle
- Cardiac pacemaker in situ

If the patient has any of the above, placement of the PICC should be avoided on that side of the patient's body where possible (Gabriel 2006).

Patient preference

When any VAD is required outside of the emergency setting, the patient should be consulted regarding their preference for the intended cannulation site. Not only will this confirm if the patient is left or right handed, ensuring the non-dominant arm is considered as the first preference, it will also allow the patient time to develop a rapport with the health professional placing the device, and thereby reduce their anxiety (Gabriel 2000).

Anaesthetic techniques

Procedures which are perceived as routine and straightforward by health professionals, e.g. cannulation, can be worrying for the patient. A clear explanation of the procedure and what to expect can go a long way in reducing anxiety for an individual patient. Where the procedure is likely to be protracted or more invasive, e.g. midline or CVAD placement, local anaesthetic agents can be used to minimise the discomfort for the patient. These can range from topical anaesthetic creams to infiltration of local anaesthetic drugs (RCN 2005, Dougherty 2006). For children, and some adults, general anaesthesia may be required.

Benefits of PICCs

PICCs have numerous benefits. Insertion early in the course of therapy is the most cost-effective use of PICCs and of health professionals' time. Overall, PICCs have reduced risks in comparison to tunnelled, non-tunnelled catheters or subcutaneously implanted ports. PICCs carry the overall lowest sepsis rate for all types of CVADs at approximately 4/1000 catheter days (Moreau *et al.* 2002). PICCs also have the advantage of placement in a variety of clinical settings including wards, outpatient clinics, and are relatively easy to insert compared to other CVADs. They can be used for a wide range of parenteral therapies as they are true CVADs, and with careful management can achieve long dwell times (www.oley.org, Dougherty 2006, Gabriel 2006).

Consent and patient information

Informed consent is the act of obtaining a patient's permission to proceed with a treatment/procedure. After an appropriate explanation of the procedure has been provided, including the risks, benefits and alternatives, the procedure may proceed. The patient should be provided with written information regarding the PICC insertion procedure, catheter management, potential complications and who to contact if they will be living with their PICC away from the hospital environment. All information must be provided in a manner consistent with the level of comprehension of the patient.

Measurements

Measurements are required to determine the length of catheter needed to reach the SVC. This will vary according to the patient's size, insertion technique and the position of the venepuncture site. If fluoroscopy is used, the length is measured either from the guidewire markings after its tip has been correctly sited in the SVC, or directly from the catheter insertion itself.

If fluoroscopic guidance is not used, measurement is achieved by the external estimate method, using a tape measure following the path of the vessels. The patient's arm should be abducted 45° from the body during this process. Using a tape measure, the measurement commences at the planned point of venepuncture, proceeding up the arm to a mid point on the clavicle and turning to reach the third intercostal space to the right of the sternum (Lum 2004). For right-sided placement, locate the first intercostal space below the clavicle, and then slide down towards the sternum. Keeping your finger on the first intercostal space, place your second finger on the second space between the ribs and third finger onto the third space; spreading the fingers as you go and staying close to the sternum. When measuring from the left, cross the sternum to reach the right side of the SVC. The distance from the left is always slightly longer since the SVC is positioned just under the right side of the sternum. This is one of the most effective methods for external measurement, but is only an estimate of the length which must be confirmed by X-ray (CXR) after placement and prior to commencing treatment. Lum (2004) studied the length of catheter in relation to body size as another means of identifying catheter length (Table 8.1).

Insertion procedures

See appendices for detail of insertion procedures.

Ensure the patient is comfortable, able to extend their arm and the bed is at the correct height for the comfort of the practitioner. Collect all the supplies needed for the procedure. PICC insertions are best performed with a team approach, i.e. one inserter and one assistant. An assistant provides an enhanced degree of safety for both the patient and the practitioner. Right-sided arm placement is preferred, due to the straighter, more

Table 8.1 Measurement guide for PICCs related to patient height.

Height	Right PICC	Left PICC
4 ft 8 in. (143 cm)	42.5 cm	46.5 cm
5 ft (153 cm)	45.5 cm	49.5 cm
5 ft 4 in. (163 cm)	48.5 cm	52.5 cm
5 ft 8 in. (173 cm)	51.5 cm	55.5 cm
6 ft (183 cm)	54.5 cm	58.5 cm
6 ft 4 in. (193 cm)	57.5 cm	61.5 cm

From 2.5 cm below antecubital fossa line.
Adapted from Lum (2004).

direct path of the vein to the SVC and lower thrombotic risk, but this may not always be possible (see assessment section) (Dougherty 2006).

Ultrasound

Clinical evidence has consistently validated ultrasound guidance as a safer method of insertion for central venous catheters (NICE 2002). Ultrasound guidance increases the success rates for central line insertion, avoiding complications and patient discomfort associated with 'blind' venepuncture (RCN 2005, Dougherty 2006). Adding ultrasound guidance to an existing PICC insertion service increases the rate of successful insertions to an average of 90% or more (RCN 2005, Dougherty 2006). Ultrasound guidance provides clear visualisation of veins and aids identification of potentially problematic anatomical issues (Dougherty 2006).

Documentation

Documentation of PICC insertion (RCN 2005, Dougherty 2006) should include:

- Insertion date and time
- Length of the catheter inserted and the external length
- Size of catheter, manufacturer, batch number
- Number of cannulation attempts and where in relation to vein location
- Any threading problems
- Flushing solution
- Securement method
- Type of dressing applied
- X-ray confirmation result
- Name of inserter
- Patient response and comments by the patient
- Document education/information given to the patient

Education

Ongoing education is crucial for all health care workers, especially in rapidly developing areas of care such as IV therapy. For all staff involved in caring for patients who have VADs in situ, basic and regular education is required to cover areas such as:

- Hand hygiene
- Adherence to aseptic care
- Update on latest guidelines, etc.
- Update on new products and their appropriate use
- Sharps safety

Patient education

Patients have a vested interest in their VADs, especially if they will be 'living with' a CVAD away from the hospital environment. They will require information/education relating to prevention of infection and gaining prompt access to an appropriate health care worker for further information about any concerns they may have relating to their device/treatment.

Power injection

Computerised tomography (CT) is increasingly used in medicine with many oncology patients having serial scans to assess tumour progression/response to treatment. Contrast is required to be injected quickly to delineate blood vessels. The pressure limit for the average PICC is 250 psi or a rate of 3–5 mL/second. Exceeding this maximum pressure/rate may result in catheter failure and/or tip displacement. PICCs designed only for CT injection (power injection) should be used (Salis 2004). Clearly, a decision needs to be made with referring clinicians before the catheter is inserted to make the choice between a conventional or power PICC, the latter is likely to be more expensive **initially but will ultimately be cost effective as the PICC can be used for a wide range of therapies/procedures.** Similar considerations apply to other catheters and ports.

Catheter rupture/damage

Rupture of a CVAD can be minimised by ensuring that high-pressure methods of drug/fluid administration are avoided, i.e. needles smaller than 21 g, syringes smaller than 10 mL (Conn 1993, RCN 2005, Dougherty 2006). Vacuumed blood collection bottles and infusion pumps should not be used without consulting the manufacturer's literature for each individual CVAD (Conn 1993, RCN 2005).

A condition known as pinch-off syndrome can occur as a result of a CVAD placed via the subclavian vein becoming compressed between the clavicle and the first rib. This can lead to fracture and migration of the catheter's tip (Dougherty 2006) (see Chapters 7 and 12).

Conclusion

PICCs are a versatile CVAD, increasing in use and popularity throughout the world. They are recognised for their low risk of complications when compared to other CVADS, ease of insertion, low infection rate and overall patient satisfaction.

However, it is crucial that all staff involved in caring for patients who have a PICC in situ, or are being considered for such a device, have the appropriate skills and knowledge. PICCs are an addition to our current range of CVADs and not a replacement.

Appendix

Needle access (21 g) for short wire introduction with sheath dilator combination for catheter threading – modified Seldinger technique

Prepare the patient

1. Apply anaesthetic as prescribed to the area of access.
2. Insert needle through skin and down to touch the top of the vein. If using ultrasound, watch for the needle track and movement as the needle moves down to the top of the vein. You should see the needlepoint touch the top of the vein and 'tent' or dimple the vein wall prior to penetration into the vein.
3. Access vein with (21 g) needle or peripheral cannula.
4. When using ultrasound, the angle of needle insertion is acute (60–90°), dependent on depth of the vein indicated by ultrasound assessment. Determine the best angle needed to touch the top of the vein directly under the ultrasound probe.
5. Observe blood return flashback.
6. Thread short wire through access device, maintaining total control of the wire at all times. Observe markings on wire to determine depth inserted. Insert approximately half the length of the wire, or 15–20 cm (short wires are generally used with this bedside procedure).
7. Remove tourniquet.
8. Remove needle access device by sliding out of the skin and off the wire, leaving wire within the vascular system.
9. Inject anaesthetic intradermally/subcutaneously into skin around the wire if not previously performed or if more needed.
10. Use blade to nick the skin and expand insertion hole. Slide blade into insertion hole about 1 cm with sharp side facing outwards dull side towards wire. Cut to one side, avoid cutting straight up.
11. Slide sheath dilator over wire and all the way into the vein using a firm twisting motion. Maintain control of the wire at all times.
12. Remove dilator by unlocking luer connector and sliding back on wire.
13. Remove the wire (sheath and wire may be removed together). Place thumb over sheath opening to reduce blood loss and prevent air emboli.
14. Thread catheter through the sheath slowly. Ask patient to turn head towards insertion site as catheter is advanced past the shoulder, into great vessels in the chest, to prevent advancement of catheter into jugular veins. Advance catheter to predetermined length on the basis of previous measurements.
15. Gently pull sheath out of skin and peel apart. Advance the catheter a little more if some of the device has pulled back with sheath removal.
16. Check for blood return through aspiration. Flush all lumens well (5–20 mL).
17. Secure the catheter and apply pressure dressing.
18. Radiographically confirm terminal PICC tip location prior to use.
19. Document procedure in patient record.

Over the needle peel away direct approach

Prepare patient as described in Section 'Insertion procedure'

1. Visualise or palpate to locate the vein of choice. Access vein using a shallow angle of insertion (15–30°). Advance the needle through the skin, dropping the angle slightly to access the vein.
2. Once blood return is achieved, drop the needle angle flat with the skin, advancing the needle a little more into the vein.
3. Advance the peel away sheath into the vein (do not break), using the needle as a slide. Remove the needle (or engage the protective device), leaving the peel away sheath in the vein.
4. Begin threading the catheter into the peel away sheath.
5. Release tourniquet.
6. Continue to slowly thread the PICC along the vein. Slow movements will reduce the risk of damage to the intima of the vein and of mechanical phlebitis. Slow advancement will also create a better opportunity for the catheter to reach the SVC rather than advancement into the vessels of the neck.
7. Ask the patient to turn their head towards the side of insertion as the catheter advances past the shoulder and into the great vessels within the chest. This will reduce the risk of the PICC advancing into the veins of the neck.
8. Complete predetermined advancement of the PICC. Pull the sheath out of the skin and peel apart swinging the wings up and down to break, then peel pulling up and out. Caution: take care not to completely dislodge the catheter during the pull and peel, a small amount of movement is acceptable with the catheter threaded again after sheath removal.
9. Check for blood return through syringe aspiration of the catheter.
10. Flush all lumens well (5–20 mL) sodium chloride 0.9% and heparinised saline.
11. Secure the catheter and apply pressure dressing.
12. Radiographically confirm SVC terminal tip location prior to infusion of medications.
13. Document in patient's record the final catheter tip position, the product code and lot number.

Needle access (21 g) for short wire introduction with sheath dilator combination for catheter threading – modified Seldinger technique

1. Prepare the patient as described in the previous steps.
2. Inject anaesthetic as needed to the area of access. Insert needle through skin and down to touch the top of the vein. If using ultrasound, watch for the needle track and movement as the needle moves down to the top of the vein. You should see the needlepoint touch the top of the vein and 'tent' or dimple the vein wall prior to penetration into the vein.
3. Access vein with (21 g) needle or peripheral cannula.
4. When using ultrasound the angle of needle insertion is acute (60–90°), dependent on depth of the vein indicated by ultrasound assessment. Determine the best angle needed to touch the top of the vein directly under the ultrasound probe.
5. Observe blood return flashback.

6. Thread short wire through access device, maintaining total control of the wire at all times. Observe markings on wire to determine depth inserted. Insert approximately half the length of the wire, or 15–20 cm (short wires are generally used with this bedside procedure).
7. Remove tourniquet.
8. Remove needle access device by sliding out of the skin and off the wire, leaving wire within the vascular system.
9. Inject anaesthetic intradermally/subcutaneously into skin around the wire if not previously performed or if more needed.
10. Use blade to nick the skin and expand insertion hole. Slide blade into insertion hole about 1 cm with sharp side facing outwards dull side towards wire. Cut to one side, avoid cutting straight up.
11. Slide sheath dilator over wire and all the way into the vein using a firm twisting motion. Maintain control of the wire at all times.
12. Remove dilator by unlocking luer connector and sliding back on wire.
13. Remove the wire (sheath and wire may be removed together). Place thumb over sheath opening to reduce blood loss and prevent air emboli.
14. Thread catheter through the sheath slowly. Ask patient to turn head towards insertion site as catheter is advanced past the shoulder, into great vessels in the chest, to prevent advancement of catheter into jugular veins. Advance catheter to predetermined length on the basis of previous measurements.
15. Gently pull sheath out of skin and peel apart. Advance the catheter a little more if some of the device has pulled back with sheath removal.
16. Check for blood return through aspiration. Flush all lumens well (5–20 mL).
17. Secure the catheter and apply pressure dressing.
18. Radiographically confirm terminal PICC tip location prior to use.
19. Document procedure in patient record.

References

Conn C (1993). The importance of syringe size when using implanted vascular access devices. *Journal of Vascular Access Network* 3:11–18.

Dougherty L (2006). Care and management. In *Central Venous Access Devices*, Dougherty L (ed.), Blackwell Publishing, Oxford, UK.

Dougherty L (2008). Peripheral venous access. In *IV Therapy in Nursing Practice*, Dougherty L, Lamb J (eds), Blackwell Publishing, Oxford, UK.

Gabriel J (1996a). Peripherally inserted central catheters: expanding UK nurses' practice. *Surgical Nurse* 5:71–77.

Gabriel J (1996b). Care and management of peripherally inserted catheters. *British Journal of Nursing* 5:594–599.

Gabriel J (2000). Care and management of peripherally inserted central catheters. In *Aspects of Cardiovascular Nursing – BJN Monograph*, Cruickshank J, Bradbury M, Ashurst S (eds), Quay Books, London, UK.

Gabriel J (2006). Vascular access. In *Nursing in Hematological Oncoclogy*, 2nd edn, Grundy M (ed.), Bailliere, Tindall, Elsevier, Edinburgh, UK.

Gabriel J (2008). Long term central venous access. In *IV Therapy in Nursing Practice*, 2nd edn, Dougherty L, Lamb J (eds), Blackwell Publishing, Oxford, UK.

Griffiths V (2007). Midline catheters: indications, complications and maintenance. *Nursing Standard* 21(22):48–57.

Hadaway L (2006). Infiltration and extravasation from vascular access devices. In *Oral presentation 20th Annual Association of Vascular Access (AVA) Conference*, Indianapolis, USA, September.

Kayley J (2003). An overview of community intravenous therapy in the United Kingdom. *Journal of Vascular Access Devices* 8:22–26.

Lum P (2004). A new formula-based measurement guide for optimal positioning of central venous catheters. *Journal of the Association for Vascular Access* 9:80–85.

Moreau N, Poole S, Murdock MA *et al.* (2002). Central venous catheters in home infusion care: outcomes analysis in 50,470 patients. *Journal of Vascular Interventional Radiology* 13(10):1009–1016.

Nakazawa N (2006). Difficult peripherally inserted central catheter (PICC) insertions. *Journal of the Association for Vascular Access* 11:124–128.

NICE (National Institute for Clinical Excellence) (2002). *Ultrasound Imaging for Central Venous Catheter Placement*. Department of Health, London, UK.

RCN (Royal College of Nursing) (2005). *Standards for Infusion Therapy*. RCN, London, UK.

Salis AI, Eclavea A, Johnson MS *et al.* (2004). Maximal flow rates possible during power injection through currently available PICCs: an in vitro study. *Journal of Vascular and Interventional Radiology* 15(3):275–281.

Schelper R (2003). The aging venous system. *Journal of the Association of Vascular Access* 8:8–10.

Chapter 9

Ultrasound-guided venous access

Andrew R. Bodenham

Introduction

The rationale for the use of ultrasound is to provide fast, reliable, safe guidance for needle placement in a vein, both for routine and difficult cases. Its use in this indication is gradually increasing as a new generation of clinicians acquire ultrasound skills and appropriate bedside machines become available. Nevertheless there is still a reluctance by some practitioners to adopt such technology.

Is there a clinical need?

Most clinicians will have seen occasional severe morbidity or mortality from central venous access, and reported complications represent only the tip of the iceberg. Most published studies quote significant complications for central venous access between 1 and 10% dependent on clinical case mix and the skill and experience of the operator (Sznajder *et al.* 1986, Mansfield *et al.* 1994, Karakitsos *et al.* 2006). Such figures are generally quoted for routine venous access, and are likely to be considerably higher for the more difficult case or novice operator. In the author's experience, most operators tend to underestimate the frequency of complications. There is good evidence that the risk of early complications is clearly related to the number of needle passes (Mansfield *et al.* 1994). Such procedural complications are well recognised and those obviously related to needle puncture are listed in Box 9.1 (see also Chapter 12).

To date, clinicians and patients have tended to accept that needle-related procedural complications are an inevitable and inherent consequence of such techniques. The widespread use of ultrasound with documented reductions in complication rates make such acceptance increasingly unsupportable. It should be appreciated that ultrasound will only help with the needle placement and give limited information on guidewire or catheter placement. It will not protect against vessel damage from dilators, catheters or

---

Box 9.1 Some procedural complications of venous access.

(Specifically related to needle damage)
Inadvertent arterial puncture
Pneumothorax
Damage to trachea, oesophagus, lymphatics
Venous tears
Venous thrombosis
Nerve damage
Increased risk of local and systemic infection

---

guidewires, but it is intuitive that accurate central placement of needle and guidewires in the correct patent vessel is fundamental to subsequent safe catheter placement.

In addition to obvious procedural complications, other issues are commonly ignored, but are likely to be significant. These include patient pain and discomfort, delayed or cancelled procedures and surgery, delayed administration of intravenous fluids/medications, complaints and medicolegal issues, and delayed discharge from hospital. Reported studies tend only to record rates of eventual catheter placement success, which may require multiple needle passes. It is likely that multiple punctures, even if eventually successful, will lead to an increased risk of subsequent venous thrombosis and catheter-related sepsis (Karakitsos *et al.* 2006).

Rationale for the use of ultrasound

The wide variability in vascular anatomy is well recognised with multiple patterns of dominant, absent, duplicate or other variant vessels (see individual chapters on specific anatomical areas). There is a wide range in patient size and shape from the neonate to the morbidly obese. Patients who have had longer-term venous access frequently have diseased vessels with thrombosis (Figure 9.1), stenosis, obstruction and venous collateral formation (see Chapters 2, 3 and 10). These factors demonstrate flaws in the concept of blind landmark-based techniques. The value of ultrasound in the recognition and management of problem cases has been documented (Hatfield and Bodenham 1999, Forauer and Glockner 2000).

Ultrasound can provide the following:

- Evidence of a large suitable patent vein. The presence of respiratory variation in vein size and antegrade flow with a normal Doppler signal suggest direct continuity with the vena cava and right atrium (Conkbayir-Isik *et al.* 2002). The presence of thrombus or a small scarred contracted vessel or multiple collaterals should prompt operators to reconsider and choose an alternative site of access. Valves are frequently seen in the proximal internal jugular, subclavian and femoral veins and should be avoided by moving the intended puncture site slightly more proximally or distally.
- An empty vein with further marked collapse in inspiration suggests hypovolaemia. Cannulation procedures may be helped by steep head down tilt (Trendelenberg position), volume loading, positive pressure ventilation, a Valsalva manoeuvre and timing

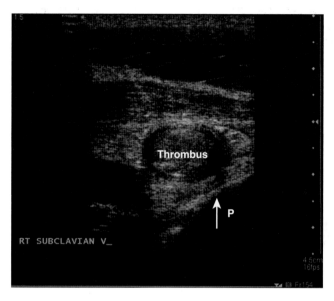

Figure 9.1 Non-compressible thrombus completely blocking the right subclavian vein; P, chest wall/pleura. Less complete thrombosis may be seen in cross section as a crescent of non-compressible echogenic material in the vein.

the vein puncture with respiration. Operators should be able to visualise when the needle has transfixed the vein to alert them to go no deeper and pull back until blood is aspirated. Sharp finer bore needles and appropriate guidewires (e.g. micropuncture kits) are helpful in such circumstances.

- Conversely, ultrasound guidance will help in cannulation of central veins in the head-up position, if required, due to brain injury or in the breathless patient with congestive cardiac failure or morbid obesity (see Chapter 3) (Brederlau *et al.* 2004).
- First pass venepuncture in most cases, into the centre of the vessel. Often in well-filled veins, only the front wall of the vessel requires puncture, avoiding transfixion, due to the improved control of the needle.
- Visualisation of collateral structures to avoid, e.g. arteries, nerves and pleura. Higher resolution devices increasingly allow identification of larger nerve bundles (Marhofer *et al.* 2005). The approach of the needle can be orientated so that the vein is not overlying the artery, pleura or other vital structures.
- Limited visualisation of needle/guidewire/catheter in the vein (Figures 9.2a–9.2c).
- Some evidence of catheter tip misplacement. The catheter can be seen if it has migrated up into the neck or to the contralateral side.

Limitations of ultrasound guidance

- Ultrasound guidance will not allow first-time users instant success. There is a definite learning curve, with some individuals finding ultrasound concepts, three-dimensional visualisation of body structures and needle guidance easier to learn than others (Sites-Brian *et al.* 2004).

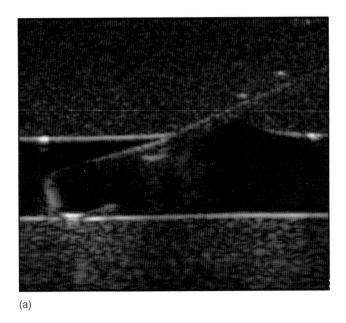

(a)

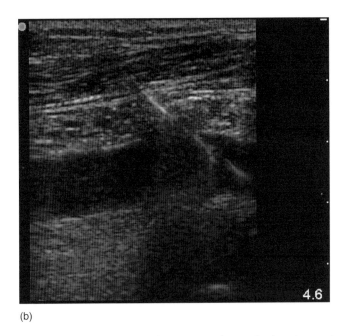

(b)

Figure 9.2 (a) Ultrasound image of a J-tipped guidewire seen in longitudinal section passing through a needle into an agar phantom with a fluid-filled central channel. (b) A guidewire is seen passing from left to right into the axillary subclavian vein. (c) A needle is seen passing from right to left into the internal jugular vein, note bright white tip of the needle. RIJV, right internal jugular vein; RCA, right carotid artery.

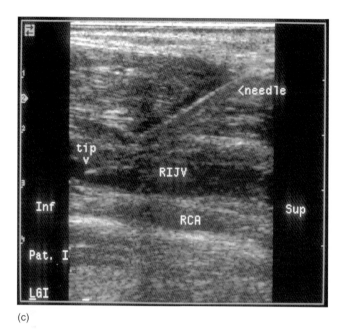

(c)

Figure 9.2 *(Continued)*

- Standard probes cannot easily visualise the inferior vena cava and right atrium due to interference from the sternum and air-filled lung. Transoesophageal echocardiography is necessary in order to visualise the inferior vena cava with ultrasound.
- Damage to other collateral structures can still occur unless operators can consistently visualise the needle tip, and guide it accurately into the target vessel. This is, in my opinion, a major limitation for many operators (Chapman *et al.* 2006). Initial correct vessel puncture may not avoid subsequent damage from guidewire, catheter or dilator insertion.

What is the evidence that ultrasound is helpful?

There have been a number of studies comparing ultrasound to so-called 'landmark techniques'. In the UK, the National Institute of Clinical Excellence (NICE) commissioned an analysis of this area of practice (NICE 2002, Hind *et al.* 2003). An analysis of all randomised trials showed that there was insufficient evidence to comment on routes other than via the internal jugular vein. For this route, the study showed the use of ultrasound provided a lower failure rate overall, and a lower failure rate on first pass of the needle. There was decreased time for cannulation, a lower frequency of complications and a potential cost savings overall. An earlier analysis showed similar findings (Randolph *et al.* 1996). NICE recommended ultrasound guidance to be used for elective cannulation of the internal jugular vein. More recent studies have clearly confirmed such findings (Karakitsos *et al.* 2006, Wigmore *et al.* 2007). Similar advantages are seen for cannulation of veins at other sites.

A number of observational studies support the use of ultrasound in patients with 'normal' and 'abnormal' anatomy. Conversely, a few case series and reports have suggested ultrasound is unhelpful or makes the frequency of complications higher. These findings maybe secondary to operator inexperience, a lack of training, restricted use of ultrasound prior to needle insertion (Hayashi and Amano 2002) or the use of inadequate devices in the more challenging case, e.g. the very small child, rather than a fundamental weakness of the technology (Grebenik *et al.* 2004). Ultrasound guidance had developed more quickly in adult practice than in paediatrics. However, similar benefits in children are starting to be realised (Chuan *et al.* 2005, Leyvi *et al.* 2005), but the size of vessels in neonates challenges current non-specialised equipment.

There are costs involved in securing ready access to ultrasound devices in all areas where vascular procedures are performed (Calvert *et al.* 2003, Scott 2003). Equally, there are costs associated with training and accreditation of a large pool of operators to perform such procedures (Bodenham 2006).

Ultrasound probe selection

Optimum visualisation of superficial vessels is obtained by using a small parts linear probe with a frequency 5 to 10 MHz. More expensive devices will have colour flow and other Doppler capabilities, which will assist in differentiation of arterial and venous blood flow, and depict direction of flow within vessels, but are unnecessary for basic use. Ultrasound features which distinguish arteries and veins are summarised in Box 9.2.

Vessels can be visualised in transverse or longitudinal planes. Size, depth, patency and flow can be assessed with ultrasound. The presence of valves, thrombus or other anatomical abnormalities can be assessed. The optimum site for venepuncture in any

---

Box 9.2 Distinguishing features of veins and arteries with ultrasound.

Real-time images are required because of dynamic changes.

Arteries
> Pulsatile,
> Resistant to compression,
> Round shape,
> Visibility improves with compression through the probe,
> Characteristic Doppler signal.

Veins
> Elliptical shape,
> Easily compressed,
> Respiratory variation in size,
> Increased size with Valsalva, or dependent position.
> Characteristic Doppler signal.

individual patient can then be decided. There are also other devices which provide an audible signal only using a Doppler probe. There is conflicting evidence for their usefulness and they are not recommended in the recent UK NICE appraisal (NICE 2002, Hind *et al.* 2003).

Applied ultrasound anatomy

Veins (see also Chapters 5–7 on individual routes of access)

Internal jugular vein

The vein lies surprisingly superficial (1–2 cm deep) and lies close (alongside or partially overlapping) to the carotid artery (see Chapter 5). However, there can be a wide variability in their relationship (Denys and Uretsky 1991), in part dependent on the orientation of the ultrasound probe. Some patients will have a dominant venous drainage on one or other side of the neck, and in occasional patients one vein will be congenitally absent. Associated structures like the thyroid and trachea are easily visualised.

Axillary/subclavian vein

Surface landmark approaches via the infraclavicular routes to the subclavian and axillary vein are well described elsewhere. The presence of the clavicle restricts ultrasound

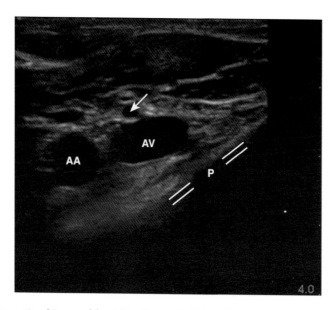

Figure 9.3 Cross-sectional image of the right axillary vein (AV), axillary artery (AA) and chest wall/pleura (P). There is a branch of the axillary artery (the thoraco-acromial artery) anterior to the vein (arrow).

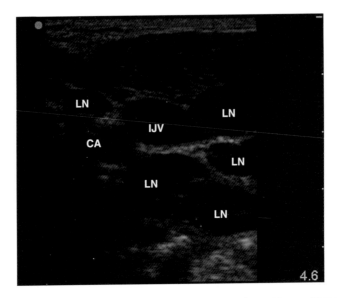

Figure 9.4 Cross-sectional image of right internal jugular vein (IJV) and carotid artery (CA) in a patient with massive lymphadenopathy from haematological malignancy. The lymph nodes (LN) resemble vessels on initial viewing but are slightly more echogenic, and have none of the other characteristics of vessels (see Figure 9.3).

visualisation of the subclavian vein in adults and the larger child. Access can be achieved by a supraclavicular approach, but it is more usual to move a short distance laterally over the deltopectoral triangle to visualise the axillary artery, vein and their branches, in particular the cephalic vein (see Figure 9.4).

The chest wall and pleura are easily visualised and identified by the characteristic appearances of ribs in transverse section and the echogenic pleura with the sliding lung sign (Galloway and Bodenham 2003). On moving further laterally, overlap of the artery and vein decreases and the chest wall and pleura falls away from the vein (a misplaced needle transfixing the vein does not hit vital structures). However, the vein becomes smaller and deeper. The brachial plexus is just cephalad to the artery and can be seen with higher resolution devices (Klaastad *et al.* 2004, Marhofer *et al.* 2005). Ultrasound offers easy access to this site except in the very obese or muscular patient, and a large clinical experience of this approach is developing (Sharma *et al.* 2004).

Femoral vein

The femoral vein is traditionally identified by palpating the artery and then directing a needle medially, assuming there is only one major vein and artery lying in a side by side position. However, the anatomy is more complex (for images, see Chapter 6). Often it is the superficial branch of the femoral artery that is most easily palpated, and the level of the inguinal ligament it difficult to identify even in thin subjects.

Traditional anatomical teaching suggests that the superficial femoral artery does not cross the femoral vein until several centimetres below the inguinal ligament, but this is not the case. Computerised tomography and ultrasound studies have shown that crossover is much higher than is commonly appreciated (Baum *et al.* 1989, Hughes *et al.* 2000). This is one reason why inadvertent arterial puncture is common via this route. In addition, the femoral vein receives several branches high in the groin notably the long saphenous vein, which may approach the size of the femoral vein at the junction. If the puncture is too high then there are risks of retroperitoneal haemorrhage if vessels are damaged.

The use of ultrasound allows accurate verification of anatomy and accurate first pass puncture of the common femoral vein immediately below the inguinal ligament. Ultrasound does not allow easy visualisation anteriorly above the inguinal ligament due to gas-filled bowel in the peritoneum. The larger vessels can be followed down into the thigh, and there have been limited reports of access via these lower routes.

Arm and leg

Deeper veins in the arm can be cannulated via ultrasound guidance even when they cannot be palpated or visualised. Techniques have been described for both short- and long-term access, in particular the use of PICC lines from the antecubital fossa (Sofocleous *et al.* 1999) or other catheters higher in the upper arm above the elbow flexure (Sandhu and Sidhu 2004). These approaches may be particularly useful in the obese patients whose superficial veins are obscured by fat or the intravenous drug abuser with thrombosed superficial veins. The leg veins can be used in a similar fashion.

More unusual routes of access

Multiple different sites of access like the inferior vena cava, portal vein, azygous system and collaterals following great vessel obstruction have been described utilising ultrasound to guide puncture, but are beyond the scope of this chapter.

Lymphatics

Lymph nodes may be mistaken for vessels as a result of their presence close to major arteries and veins (Figure 9.4). Lymph nodes can be easily visualised with ultrasound as round structures with low echogenicity. They do not pulsate, or cycle in size with respiration and are not easily compressible. Scanning along the vascular trunks will demonstrate the characteristic shape of nodes. Larger lymphatic vessels are visible with ultrasound and are likely to be difficult to distinguish from veins except by the lack of a clear Doppler signal (Zironi *et al.* 1995).

Practicalities of vascular access utilising ultrasound

Check for the presence of an appropriate vessel with ultrasound before starting.

Transducer and display set-up

Touch one side of the probe and observe the image to allow orientation. An orientation marker is usually present on the side of the transducer corresponding to a marker on

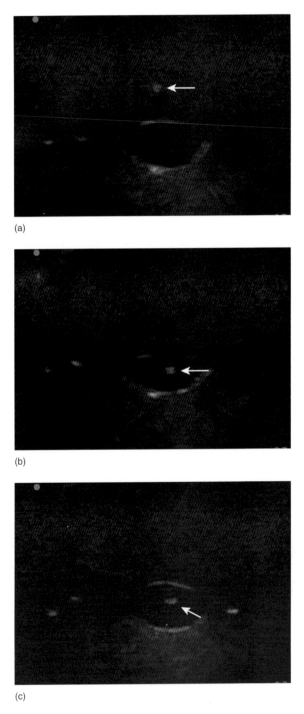

(a)

(b)

(c)

Figure 9.5 A needle is guided into an agar phantom with a fluid filled cavity to resemble a vein seen in cross section with ultrasound. (a) As the needle tip passes into the beam of the ultrasound, a white dot is seen (small arrow). (b) The angle of the needle is steepened and the needle tip is seen to approach and indent the anterior wall of the cavity, but the wall is not yet penetrated. (c) With further advancement, the needle tip (white dot) is seen in its lumen. Correct position is confirmed by free aspiration of fluid.

the display. One needs to assure that the marker is in agreement with the displayed orientation. If not then the transducer should be rotated 180°. Adjust the depth to ensure that structures are visualised in the centre of the screen. Alter the gain to create a relatively dark image that allows discrimination of the white dots generated by the needle. Use sterile ultrasound gel inside and outside the protective sterile sheath.

Position the ultrasound display at eye level on the opposite side of the patient to the operator. Place the probe lightly on the skin (veins will collapse easily). Choose a site and probe orientation where the vein lies side by side with the artery (rather than anterior to it) as the vein will often need to be transfixed to puncture its anterior wall. If the vein is transfixed, successful aspiration then occurs on gentle withdrawal of the needle.

Guidance techniques

Injected local anaesthetic will enhance visualisation of deep structures providing no air bubbles are injected. It can be injected before starting or under ultrasound guidance.

Needles can be guided through tissues directly and indirectly.

Indirect ultrasound guidance involves the identification of a patent non-diseased vessel prior to puncture. The skin is marked and an estimate is taken of the angle and depth of the needle course. This technique whilst helpful to identify blocked or absent veins cannot be recommended as collateral structures may still be hit if the approach of the needle is not correct and operators may not realise they have transfixed the vein.

Direct ultrasound guidance involves the use of ultrasound to visualise the needle in real-time. There are two techniques – the use of needle guides and free-hand puncture. An appreciation of the appearances of needles crossing the ultrasound beam in the longitudinal (long axis) and transverse (short axis) is required (Figures 9.2c and 9.5). Some needles are specifically designed to be more visible with ultrasound (Figures 9.6a and 9.6b).

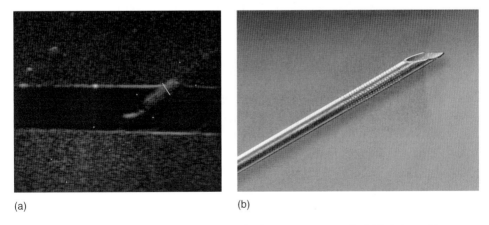

(a)   (b)

Figure 9.6 (a) EchoTip needle (Cook) seen in longitudinal section entering a fluid-filled channel in an agar phantom trainer for vascular access procedures. A needle guidance system is in use with electronic markers (white dots) showing the projected path of the needle (SonoSite Titan device). (b) Magnified image of the Echotip needle showing the machined surface just proximal to the tip.

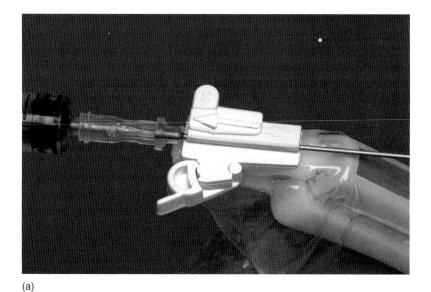

(a)

(b)

Figure 9.7 (a) A detachable single use sterile needle guide for long-axis needle insertion under ultrasound guidance. The needle follows a predetermined path as shown. (b) Single-use sterile needle guide for short-axis insertion, there are different angle guides in which the needle tip crosses the ultrasound beam at a predetermined depth. Both attached to Sonosite linear probes with a sterile plastic ultrasound cover.

Needle guides direct the needle in a predetermined direction to various depths from the transducer surface, depending on the selected angle of the guide (Figure 9.7). Guides vary and may be fixed or detachable from the transducer. They may be orientated to guide the needle in the short or long axis of the probe. Guidance lines generated on the display show the projected path of the needle (Figure 9.6). The probe is adjusted so the target vessel lies within the guidance lines and the depth assessed. The probe is held still, the needle clamped in the guide and passed through it into the tissues either to a predetermined depth or until the needle tip is positioned in the vessel.

For free-hand puncture, the needle is held with one hand and the transducer with the other. Using needle guidance techniques (see below), the needle is guided into the vein. This approach provides greater flexibility without having to use secondary instruments and allows for subtle compensatory adjustments.

Needle visualisation

This a potential weakness of many operators who have no difficulty in visualising the target vessel but fail to understand needle-tip visualisation and hence still risk needle damage during insertion procedures (Chapman *et al.* 2006).

Short-axis approach

The needle is inserted at a shallow angle until the tip (a white dot) enters the ultrasound beam. It is then withdrawn slightly, realigned more steeply and advanced until seen again in a deeper position. This sequence is repeated, correcting the insertion direction, to approach and puncture the vessel centrally (Figure 9.5). Because this approach gives poorer visualisation of the needle (the needle tip may be mistaken for the needle shaft), the position of the needle tip may need to be repeatedly re-established by either rocking the transducer or re-aligning the needle in a more vertical plane. Experienced operators will combine both techniques with small movements of the tip to verify its position. A needle passing through the ultrasound beam in short axis produces an acoustic shadow, seen as a black line passing to the base of the image.

Long-axis approach

This allows better needle visualisation if the needle is kept relatively perpendicular to the ultrasound beam (Figure 9.6). As the needle gets steeper, the image quality deteriorates. Practice is required to keep the needle and the target vessel precisely within the ultrasound beam. Novices may find this method more difficult than the short-axis approach (Blaivas *et al.* 2003, Milling *et al.* 2005).

Verification of needle-tip placement

The vein wall may occlude the needle tip, which appears to lie within the vessel lumen on ultrasound. Irrespective of the techniques used, verification of the needle-tip placement is required by either aspirating blood or noting the vein to reopen following collapse due to the pressure of the advancing needle. The needle tip may require further fine adjustment to allow passage of the guidewire, as traditionally learnt with conventional surface landmark-based techniques.

Conclusion

Ultrasound guidance is a useful technique to aid venous access. It is effective in the routine and difficult cases, improves the success rates of cannulation and reduces complications. Orientation of the ultrasound probe and needle is a skill that takes some practice, but the time spent understanding and practicing the technique will be repaid many times over when performing invasive procedures.

References

Baum PA, Matsumoto AH, Teitelbaum GP *et al.* (1989). Anatomic relationship between the common femoral artery and vein: CT evaluation and clinical significance. *Radiology* 173:775–777.

Blaivas M, Brannam L, Fernandez E (2003). Short-axis versus long-axis approaches for teaching ultrasound-guided vascular access on a new inanimate model. *Academic Emergency Medicine* 10:1307–1311.

Bodenham A (2006). Editorial II: ultrasound imaging by anaesthetists: training and accreditation issues. *British Journal of Anaesthesia* 96:414–417.

Brederlau J, Greim C, Schwemmer U *et al.* (2004). Ultrasound-guided cannulation of the internal jugular vein in critically ill patients positioned in 30 degrees dorsal elevation. *European Journal of Anaesthesiology* 21:684–687.

Calvert N, Hind D, McWilliams RG *et al.* (2003). The effectiveness and cost effectiveness of ultrasound locating devices for central venous access: a systematic review and economic evaluation. *Health Technology Assessment* 7:1–84.

Chapman GA, Johnson D, Bodenham AR (2006). Visualisation of needle position using ultrasonography. *Anaesthesia* 61:148–158.

Chuan WX, Wei W, Yu L (2005). A randomised controlled study of ultrasound prelocation vs anatomical landmark guided cannulation of the internal jugular vein in infants and children. *Pediatric Anaesthesia* 15:733–738.

Conkbayir I, Men S, Yanik B *et al.* (2002). Color Doppler sonographic finding of retrograde jugular venous flow as a sign of innominate vein obstruction. *Journal of Clinical Ultrasound* 30:392–398.

Denys BG, Uretsky BF (1991). Anatomical variation of the internal jugular vein. *Critical Care Medicine* 19:1516–1519.

Forauer AR, Glockner JF (2000). Importance of US findings in planning jugular vein haemodialysis catheter placements. *Journal of Vascular and Interventional Radiology* 11:233–238.

Galloway S, Bodenham A (2003). Ultrasound imaging of the axillary vein–anatomical basis for central venous access. *British Journal of Anaesthesia* 90:589–595.

Grebenik CR, Boyce A, Sinclair ME *et al.* (2004). NICE guidelines for central venous catheterization in children. Is the evidence base sufficient? *British Journal of Anaesthesia* 92:827–830.

Hatfield A, Bodenham A (1999). Portable ultrasound for difficult central venous access. *British Journal of Anaesthesia* 82:822–826.

Hayashi H, Amano M (2002). Does ultrasound imaging before puncture facilitate internal jugular vein cannulation? Prospective randomized comparison with landmark-guided puncture in ventilated patients. *Journal of Cardiothoracic and Vascular Anesthesia* 16:572–575.

Hind D, Calvert N, McWilliams R *et al.* (2003). Ultrasonic locating devices for central venous cannulation: meta-analysis. *BMJ* 327:361.

Hughes P, Scott C, Bodenham A (2000). Ultrasonography of the femoral veins, implications for vascular access. *Anaesthesia* 55:1199–1202.

Karakitsos D, Labropoulos N, De Groot E, *et al.* (2006). Real-time ultrasound guided catheterization of the internal jugular vein a prospective randomized comparison to the landmark technique in critical care patients. *Critical Care* 10:R162.

Klaastad Ø, Smith H-J, Smedby O *et al.* (2004). A novel infraclavicular brachial plexus block: the lateral and sagittal technique, developed by magnetic resonance imaging studies. *Anesthesia and Analgesia* 98:252–256.

Leyvi G, Taylor D, Reith E *et al.* (2005). Utility of ultrasound-guided central venous cannulation in pediatric surgical patients: a clinical series. *Pediatric Anesthesia* 15:953–958.

Mansfield PF, Hohn DC, Fornage BD *et al.* (1994). Complications and failures of subclavian-vein catheterization. *New England Journal of Medicine* 331:1735–1738.

Marhofer P, Greher M, Kapral S (2005). Ultrasound guidance in regional anaesthesia. *British Journal of Anaesthesia* 94:7–17.

Milling TJ, Rose J, Briggs WM *et al.* (2005). Randomised controlled clinical trial of point of care limited ultrasonography assistance of central venous cannulation. The third sonography outcomes assessment program (SOAP-3) trial. *Critical Care Medicine* 33:1764–1769.

NICE (National Institute for Clinical Excellence) (2002) *Guidance on the Use of Ultrasound Locating Devices for Central Venous Catheters.* NICE technology appraisal, No. 49, London, UK.

Randolph AG, Cook DJ, Gonzales CA *et al.* (1996). Ultrasound guidance for placement of central venous catheters: a meta-analysis of the literature. *Critical Care Medicine* 24:2053–2058.

Sandhu NS, Sidhu DS (2004). Mid arm approach to basilic and cephalic vein using ultrasound guidance. *British Journal of Anaesthesia* 93:292–294.

Scott DHT (2003). Editorial II: its NICE to see in the dark. *British Journal of Anaesthesia* 90:269–272.

Sharma A, Bodenham AR, Mallick A (2004). Ultrasound-guided infraclavicular axillary vein cannulation for central venous access. *British Journal of Anaesthesia* 93:188–192.

Sites-Brian D, Gallagher JD, Cravero J *et al.* (2004). Learning curve associated with a simulated ultrasound-guided interventional task by inexperienced anesthesia residents. *Regional Anesthesia and Pain Medicine* 29:544–548.

Sofocleous CT, Schur I, Cooper SG *et al.* (1999). Sonographically guided placement of peripherally inserted central venous catheters. *American Journal of Roentgenology* 170:1613–1616.

Sznajder JI, Zveibil FR, Bitterman H *et al.* (1986). Central vein catheterization. Failure and complication rates by three percutaneous approaches. *Archives of Internal Medicine* 146:259–261.

Wigmore TJ, Smythe JF, Hacking MB *et al.* (2007). Effect of the implementation of NICE guidelines for ultrasound guidance on the complication rates associated with central venous catheter placement in patients presenting for routine surgery in a tertiary referral centre. *British Journal of Anaesthesia* 99:662–665.

Zironi G, Cavalli G, Casali A *et al.* (1995). Sonographic assessment of the distal end of the thoracic duct in healthy volunteers and patients with portal hypertension. *American Journal of Radiology* 165:863–866.

Chapter 10

The role of diagnostic and interventional radiology in the placement and management of central venous catheters

Dinuke R. Warakaulle and Jane Phillips-Hughes

Introduction

The traditional role of radiologists in the management of central venous catheters (CVCs) has been to document their position following placement and to perform appropriate imaging in the event of complications arising from CVC placement. However, the relatively recent development of the subspecialty of interventional radiology has allowed radiologists to play an increasingly important part in the placement of CVCs and in the treatment of complications of long-term venous access.

Imaging modalities

(1) Plain radiographs are used to confirm CVC position and to detect pneumothorax, haemothorax or effusion development following placement. Clinicians involved with insertions of CVCs should be aware of the limitations of such imaging. The anatomical proximity of major arteries, veins and pleura in the neck and chest may cause difficulties, and it may not be possible to reliably state whether the distal section of a catheter is in an artery, vein, pleura or mediastinum in the chest from a plain PA chest X-ray, hence the often guarded statements in radiology reports. Such imaging is used primarily to check that a catheter has passed centrally into

a reasonable position where the superior vena cava (SVC) approximately lies, it is not kinked and there are no other procedural complications. Malposition may be more obvious in the aorta if the catheter has passed into the arch or descending left side, rather than in the ascending aorta. In cases of doubt, further imaging is required. Outside radiology areas, measurements of pressures or analysis of oxygen saturations of aspirated blood are helpful.

(2) Direct venography is performed by injecting iodinated contrast medium into a peripheral vein (typically in the antecubital fossa or forearm) whilst obtaining fluoroscopic images. Simultaneous injections into both arms are commonly performed. This allows assessment of the peripheral arm veins as well as the axillary, subclavian and brachiocephalic veins and the SVC. The inferior vena cava (IVC) can be assessed by injecting contrast medium into a common femoral vein, or by placing a catheter into it via the common femoral or internal jugular vein.

(3) Ultrasound can be used to assess the jugular, common femoral and distal subclavian veins and the arm veins. It is also used to guide venous punctures.

(4) Fluoroscopy is used during CVC placement to guidewires and catheters and to confirm appropriate line position.

(5) Computed tomographic (CT) and magnetic resonance (MR) imaging are cross-sectional imaging modalities that can provide information about the central veins.

(6) Linograms are performed by injecting iodinated contrast medium into the CVC whilst obtaining fluoroscopic images. These studies are used to assess line patency, line position, and to detect complications such as the development of fibrin sheaths.

Imaging venous anatomy

The anatomy of the venous system relevant to CVC placement at individual sites is detailed elsewhere in this book. Routine imaging is not performed prior to CVC placement. Relatively common anatomical variations may therefore cause confusion when plain radiographs are obtained following CVC placement without image guidance.

Bilateral SVCs are present in 0.3% of the population. The left-sided SVC most commonly drains into an enlarged coronary sinus, and the left brachiocephalic vein is absent in 65% of cases (Dähnert 1999). A CVC placed via a left subclavian or jugular venous approach would therefore have an unusual mediastinal course on a plain radiograph (Figure 10.1).

A duplicated IVC is found in 0.2–3% of the population, with the left-sided IVC draining into the left renal vein (Dähnert 1999). A CVC placed via a left common femoral venous approach would then be projected to the left of the midline on a plain radiograph. A transposed, or solitary left-sided IVC is found in 0.2–0.5% of the population (Dähnert 1999).

Imaging of the central veins may be performed in patients with a previous history of long-term or difficult venous access, to plan an approach for new CVC placement or to manage complications of previous access. Examples are shown in Figures 2.6 and 2.7, where venography was performed in patients who had previous long-term access via upper body veins. The studies demonstrate occlusion of the great veins, with venous return occurring via numerous collaterals.

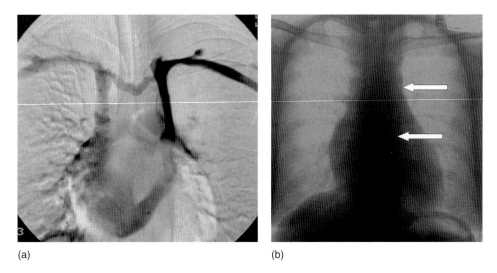

(a)   (b)

Figure 10.1 A digital subtraction venographic image (a) demonstrates bilateral SVCs. There is a connection between the two representing a left brachiocephalic remnant. The left side is blacker due to injections being slightly asynchronous. The left SVC drains to the right heart by an enlarged coronary sinus. A plain radiograph (b) obtained after CVC placement via a left internal jugular venous approach shows the catheter (arrows) passing via the left-sided SVC into the coronary sinus. The CVC functioned normally.

Image-guided CVC placement

A detailed discussion of CVC placement using anatomical landmarks and ultrasound is found elsewhere in this book, and this section is restricted to describing the utility of image guidance in the various steps involved in performing this procedure.

Venous puncture

The right internal jugular vein is our preferred puncture site for the placement of CVCs. This vein, due to its superficial location, is usually amenable to ultrasound-guided puncture. A high frequency (7–10 MHz) linear transducer is used. The vein is punctured where it lies lateral to the common carotid artery (Figures 10.2a and 10.2b). As the vein may collapse when puncture is attempted, a 'through and through' puncture – where the vein is transfixed by the needle, followed by gradual needle withdrawal until the aspiration of blood confirms the intraluminal position of the needle tip – is sometimes required. If this is performed lateral to the common carotid artery, the risk of inadvertent arterial puncture can be minimised. Colour flow and continuous wave Doppler ultrasound can be used to differentiate arteries from veins in the event of uncertainty. The pulsatile flow within an artery is distinct from the more continuous intravenous flow (Figure 10.3).

The arm veins which may be used for peripherally inserted central catheter (PICC) placement and the common femoral veins are also usually readily visible on ultrasound. The subclavian vein can also be punctured under ultrasound guidance in most patients (Figure 10.4).

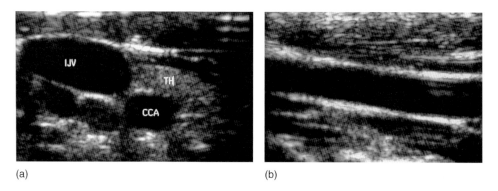

(a)   (b)

Figure 10.2 Axial (a) and longitudinal (b) ultrasound images of the right internal jugular vein. CCA, right common carotid artery; IJV, right internal jugular vein; TH, right thyroid lobe.

Ultrasound-guided venous puncture has been recognised as a safe and reliable technique which minimises the risk of inadvertent arterial puncture (Hind *et al.* 2003). The National Institute for Clinical Excellence recommends ultrasound guidance as the preferred method of CVC insertion into the internal jugular vein and also recommends consideration of ultrasound guidance for CVC placement in most clinical circumstances (National Institute for Clinical Excellence 2002).

Venous puncture is usually carried out with a one-part, 19 gauge needle which accommodates a 0.035 in. guidewire. Micropuncture sets comprising a 22 gauge needle and 0.018 in. guidewire have a theoretically lower risk of causing significant haemorrhage

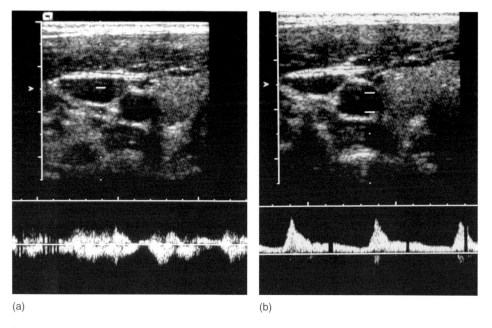

(a)   (b)

Figure 10.3 Continuous Doppler flow within the internal jugular vein (a) differs from the pulastile flow seen in the common carotid artery (b).

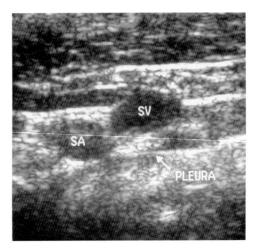

Figure 10.4 Ultrasound image of the subclavian vein (SV) and artery (SA). The proximity of these vessels to the pleural surface is demonstrated.

or pneumothorax due to inadvertent arterial or pleural puncture. However, we do not use them routinely in our practice as they increase the number of steps in the procedure and incur an additional cost.

Guidewire placement

A standard 0.035 in. guidewire is passed through the needle into the vein. Fluoroscopy is used to confirm wire position. Occasionally, the wire may not pass easily into the vein due to vessel tortuosity or because the needle tip lies against the vessel wall. An injection of contrast medium can be used to obtain a 'roadmap' (Figure 10.5a). This can be used to guide appropriate manipulation of the needle and wire (Figure 10.5b). A floppy-tipped guidewire may also be useful in this situation. If the guidewire loops within the right atrium (Figure 10.5c), it can be manipulated into the IVC by asking the patient to breathe in deeply while the guidewire is advanced, or by passing a general-purpose catheter over the guidewire to aid manipulation.

Positioning of the guidewire in the IVC (Figure 10.5d) results in a stable wire position, and also confirms its intravenous location, as a wire inadvertently inserted via an artery into the ascending aorta cannot pass below the diaphragm (Jackson and Cockburn 1996).

Measuring the CVC

Many catheter types (e.g. Hickman catheters) have to be cut to an appropriate length so that their tips lie within the SVC. This is achieved by laying the catheter externally on the patient's anterior chest wall along the line of the guidewire using fluoroscopy. A metal marker is used to measure the appropriate length of the catheter (Figure 10.5e). A more accurate technique is to place the tip of guidewire in desired position and measure the length of a marked guidewire or calculate by subtracting measured external portion from total length of guidewire.

Inserting the CVC

The peel-away sheath through which the CVC passes, or the catheter itself, is inserted over the guidewire. As there is a straight course from the right internal jugular vein into the SVC, fluoroscopic guidance is not required if this vein has been used for access. However, fluoroscopic guidance is required if the sheath is introduced via the left internal jugular or a subclavian venous approach. Once the sheath enters the vein through the puncture site, the inner dilator can be held back whilst the sheath is advanced to minimise the risk of perforation. Fluoroscopy is then used to confirm appropriate positioning of the CVC tip following placement (Figure 10.5f). The tip should ideally lie within the proximal SVC.

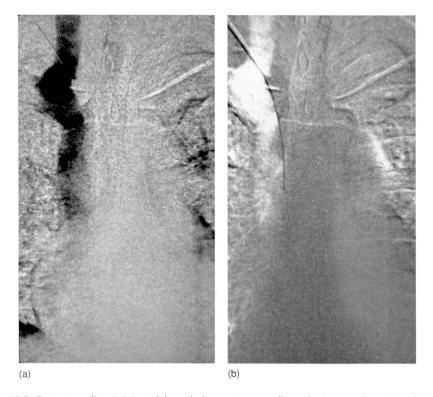

(a)   (b)

Figure 10.5 Contrast medium is injected through the puncture needle to obtain a 'roadmap' (a), which is used to guide manipulation of the wire into the SVC (b). The wire may loop within the right atrium (c), requiring manipulation into the IVC. Passage of the guidewire below the hemidiaphragm (d) confirms its position within the IVC. The CVC (arrows) is cut to an appropriate length using fluoroscopy (e). Line tip position is confirmed following the procedure (f).

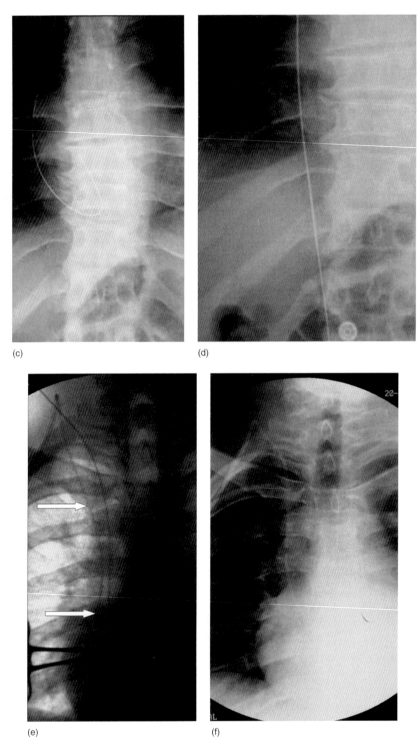

(c)

(d)

(e)

(f)

Figure 10.5 *(Continued)*

Management of CVC-related complications: the radiologist's role

The imaging modalities described above are widely used to diagnose CVC-related complications. However, interventional radiologists are increasingly involved in the management of these clinical problems, as outlined below.

Inadvertent arterial access

Inadvertent arterial puncture rates during CVC insertion as high as 8% have been reported (Wisborg *et al*. 1991). Serious complications such as the development of pseudoaneurysms, arteriovenous fistulas, local haematoma or haemothorax are more likely following arterial puncture rather than arterial catheterisation alone. The traditional management of these complications has been surgical following diagnostic angiography. However, the increasing availability of a range of percutaneous arterial closure devices for use to secure haemostasis after diagnostic and interventional vascular procedures has allowed interventional radiologists to remove CVCs placed intra-arterially over guidewires, and then closes the entry site with closure devices (Wallace and Ahrar 2001). However, arterial injury following inadvertent CVC placement may require other radiological procedures such as balloon tamponade and/or stent graft insertion (Nicholson *et al*. 2004).

Malpositioned CVCs

Incorrect placement of the CVC tip is the commonest cause of early catheter malfunction, and is more likely if insertion is performed without image guidance and in patients with multiple catheter placements. CVCs placed via the upper limb, axillary or subclavian veins are commonly malpositioned within the internal jugular vein or contralateral brachiocephalic vein. CVC tips may also be located in the azygous or superior intercostals veins. CVCs placed via the femoral veins may lie with their tips in the renal veins. This malpositioning is usually discovered on plain radiographs taken after CVC placement (Boardman and Hughes 1998).

Several methods of repositioning such catheters have been described:

(a) Forceful injection of saline or contrast into the CVC
(b) Direct manipulation by passing a guidewire through the catheter
(c) Trans femoral manipulation using angiographic catheters (Figure 10.6)
(d) Transfemoral manipulation using loop snares (Figure 10.7)

Displaced CVCs

CVCs can be displaced through vessel walls into adjacent structures. Figure 10.8 demonstrates a CVC placed via a left subclavian vein approach which passes through the SVC into the mediastinum. The catheter was placed without radiological guidance, and may have partially perforated the SVC at the time of placement. The large pleural effusions seen on the axial CT image were thought to have occurred as a result of subsequent

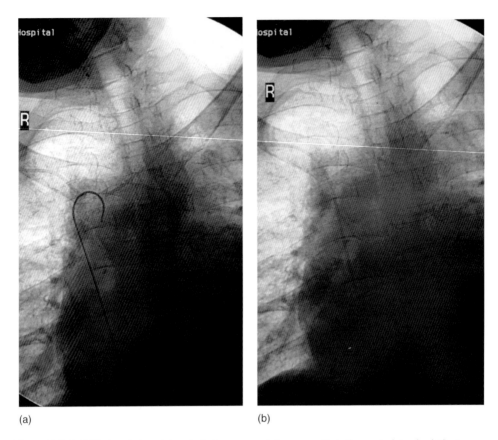

(a)   (b)

Figure 10.6 A CVC placed via a right subclavian approach has passed into the contralateral subclavian vein. An angiographic pigtail catheter inserted via a femoral venous approach (a) was used to reposition the CVC into a satisfactory position (b).

partial extravasation of chemotherapy administered through the catheter. The CVC was carefully withdrawn over a guidewire.

Fractured CVCs

Mechanical problems such as catheter kinking and compression usually require catheter replacement to restore function. Subclavian CVCs may be compressed due to entrapment by the subclavius muscle–costoclavicular ligament complex as the catheter passes beneath the clavicle. This 'pinch-off' sign is associated with CVC fracture, and if seen, should prompt catheter replacement (Boardman and Hughes 1998) (see Chapter 7).

Dislodged CVC fragments can also be retrieved percutaenously by interventional radiologists using loop snares, tip-deflecting wires, wire baskets, graspers and biopsy forceps. However, surgical arteriotomy or venotomy may be required for final removal, particularly in the case of large calibre catheter fragments (Jackson and Cockburn1996).

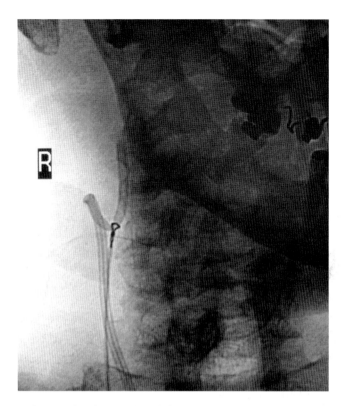

Figure 10.7 The tip of a CVC placed via a right subclavian approach is seen in the right internal jugular vein. A loop snare has been used to grasp the distal end of the catheter to allow successful repositioning.

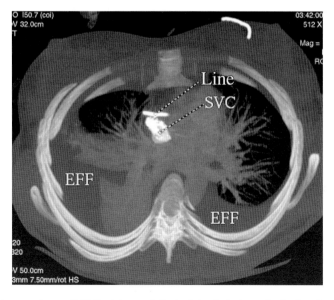

Figure 10.8 CT images show a CVC (line) inserted via the left subclavian vein displaced outside the SVC into the mediastinum. EFF, bilateral pleural effusions.

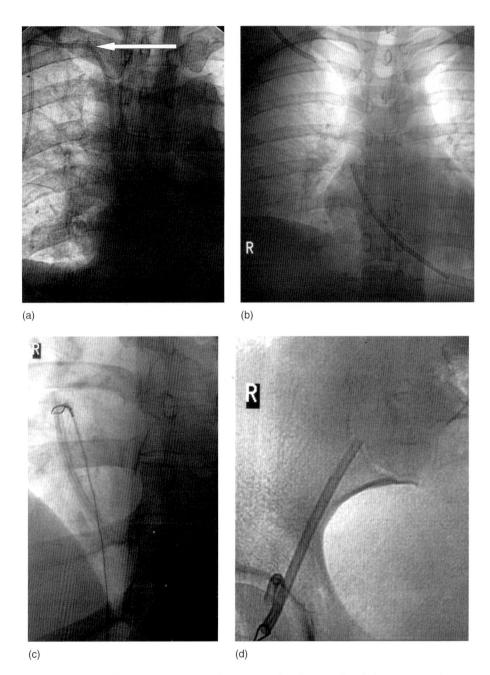

(a)   (b)

(c)   (d)

Figure 10.9 A 'pinch-off' sign (arrow) is seen where a CVC placed via a right subclavian approach passes beneath the clavicle (a). A subsequent image (b) shows fracture of the CVC at this point, with the distal fragment lodged across the tricuspid valve. The fragment was grasped with a loop snare via a femoral venous approach (c) and successfully retrieved (d).

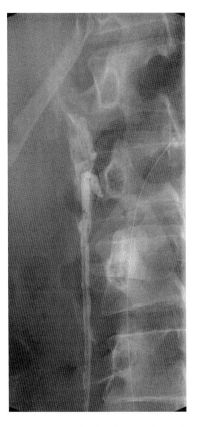

Figure 10.10 Linogram image demonstrates a fibrin sheath around the distal end of a CVC inserted via a right common femoral vein approach. Injected contrast is flowing back between the distal end of the catheter and the fibrin sheath and passes into the vein lumen.

An example of CVC 'pinch-off' with subsequent fracture is illustrated in Figure 10.9. A patient with a right subclavian CVC was noted to have catheter 'pinch-off' on a chest radiograph. However, the CVC was left in situ. The patient represented with palpitations. A repeat radiograph demonstrated CVC fracture, with the distal fragment lodged across the tricuspid valve. This was successfully retrieved via a femoral approach using a loop snare.

Fibrin sheaths

Fibrin sheath formation at the tip of a CVC can cause dysfunction. This can usually be diagnosed by performing a linogram. Fluoroscopic images are acquired at a high frame rate, while injecting contrast medium gently through the catheter. The characteristic findings include a small filling defect related to the exit port, lack of an immediate jet of contrast flowing towards the right atrium and reflux of contrast along the proximal shaft of the catheter (Figure 10.10). Fibrin sheaths can be treated by instilling a thrombolytic agent into the catheter. If this fails, the sheath can be stripped with a loop snare or disrupted with a guidewire (Boardman and Hughes 1998).

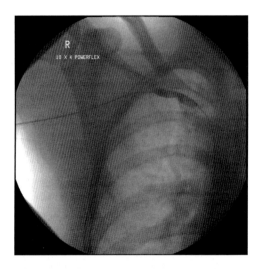

Figure 10.11 Balloon angioplasty of a stenosed right axillay vein following long-term venous access.

CVC-related venous thrombosis, stenosis and occlusion

Long-term CVC placement can result in irritation of the vein wall, leading to neointimal hyperplasia, stenosis and occlusion. Venous stenoses and occlusions may also be sequelae of catheter-related thrombosis.

Radiologists have an important role in diagnosing venous pathology related to CVC placement. Ultrasound, venography, linograms, CT and MR imaging can all be useful in this situation. The availability of hydrophilic guidewires, low-profile angioplasty balloons and flexible intravascular stents has allowed interventional radiologists to recanalise severe stenoses and even chronic total occlusions (Blum 1999). Figure 10.11 demonstrates an example; in this case, the right axillary vein was dilated with a balloon inserted via the arm, with subsequent CVC placement through the dilated vein (see also Figure 11.5).

The case shown in Figure 10.12 is an example of the varied techniques used by interventional radiologists to re-establish venous patency following CVC-related thrombosis. The patient who had a history of difficult venous access had a left subclavian CVC attached to an implantable port. The CVC was used for long-term total parenteral nutrition. The patient presented with CVC dysfunction and swelling of the face and neck. A CT scan was performed, and showed thrombotic occlusion of the SVC (similar image shown in Figure 2.4). Access was obtained via the left brachial vein, and a loop snare was used to pull the tip of the CVC back into the left axillary vein (Figure 10.12a). A mechanical thrombectomy device was then passed into the SVC and used to fragment the thrombus. This resulted in partial recanalisation of the vein. A specialised catheter with multiple side holes and an occludable end hole was then placed into the SVC to allow targeted delivery of a thrombolytic agent (recombinant tissue plasminogen activator). Following infusion of the thrombolytic agent, there was further improvement of SVC patency, although some residual clot was seen at venography. The CVC tip

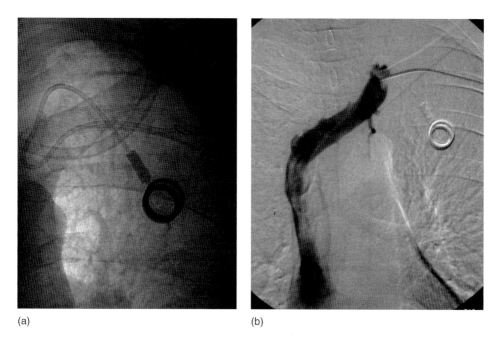

(a)   (b)

Figure 10.12 An implantable central venous port had been inserted via the left subclavian vein. (a) The venous section of the catheter was pulled back into the left axillary vein using a loop snare via a left brachial vein approach. (b) A digital subtraction venogram image taken after mechanical thrombectomy and catheter-directed thrombolysis show partial re-establishment of patency of the SVC, although there is still some residual thrombus. The catheter tip has been repositioned into the SVC. (Images provided by Dr P. Boardman, Consultant Interventional Radiologist, John Radcliffe Hospital, Oxford.)

was then snared from a right common femoral venous approach and repositioned in to the SVC (Figure 10.12b). Following this procedure, the patient's clinical symptoms improved, and CVC function was restored.

Patients with difficult venous access

Multiple previous CVC placement as well as other causes of venous stenosis and occlusion such as long-tern haemodialysis can cause difficulty when venous access is required. The commonly used routes for CVC placement may no longer be available in these patients. Interventional radiologists can place catheters into the IVC either by direct puncture under image guidance or via the hepatic veins. Patients with central venous occlusions often develop collateral veins, and these can then be used for access. Potential sites include veins in the lumbar and cervicothoracic plexuses and branches of the azygous, hemiazygous and intercostals veins (Blum 1999).

Conclusion

Radiology should play an integral part in the placement and management of CVCs. A combination of ultrasound and fluoroscopic guidance aids venous access and line placement, particularly in cases where the venous anatomy is altered or anomalous. Furthermore, various interventional radiological techniques can prolong the life of a catheter failing due to fibrin sheath formation or correct malposition of the line, preventing unnecessary line replacement.

Finally, when all conventional routes have been exhausted, radiological guidance can provide access to alternative insertion sites without resource to surgery.

References

Blum AS (1999). The role of the interventional radiologist in central venous access. *Journal of Intravenous Nursing* 22:S32–S39.

Boardman P, Hughes JP (1998). Radiological evaluation and management of malfunctioning central venous catheters. *Clinical Radiology* 53:10–16.

Dähnert W (1999). *Radiology Review Manual*, 4th edn. Williams & Wilkins, Baltimore, MD.

Hind D, Calvert N, McWilliams R *et al.* (2003). Ultrasonic locating devices for central venous cannulation: meta-analysis. *British Medical Journal* 327:361.

Jackson J, Cockburn J (1996). Venous access. In *Interventional Radiology: A Practical Guide*, 1st edn, Watkinson A, Adams A (eds), Radcliffe Medical Press, Oxford, UK.

National Institute for Clinical Excellence (2002) Guidance on the use of ultrasound locating devices for central venous catheters. Technical appraisal guidance No. 49. National Institute for Clinical Excellence, London, UK.

Nicholson T, Ettles D, Robinson G (2004). Managing inadvertent arterial catheterization during central venous access procedures. *Cardiovascular and Interventional Radiology* 27:21–25.

Wallace MJ, Ahrar K (2001). Percutaneous closure of a subclavian artery injury after inadvertent catheterization. *Journal of Vascular and Interventional Radiology*, 12:1227–1230.

Wisborg T, Flaatten H, Koller ME (1991). Percutaneous placement of permanent central venous catheters: experience with 200 catheters. *Acta Anaesthesiologica Scandinavica*. 35:49–51.

Chapter 11

Problems and practical solutions during insertion of catheters

Cathy Hartley-Jones

This chapter considers common problems encountered when attempting to insert central vascular access devices (CVAD). Insertion of a peripherally inserted central catheter (PICC) or central venous catheter (CVC) – temporary or tunnelled, using either a blind subclavian approach or an internal jugular approach under ultrasound guidance is considered. A thorough assessment and examination of the patient prior to the procedure is essential to avoid or reduce common problems. Suggestions are included to prevent the occurrence of these problems, as well as advice on management of problems should they be encountered. More significant complications are addressed in Chapter 12.

Needlephobia

An increasing number of patients are needlephobic, usually due to repeated exposure to needle pricks or a bad experience during previous venous access attempts.

Unfortunately, by the time one is faced with a needlephobic patient, prevention is too late. The insertion of a long-term CVAD may help to curtail this fear and alleviate the patient's anxiety. The best way to deal with a needlephobic patient is to try and obtain their trust through honesty and plenty of reassurance. When performing the procedure, they must be warned when to expect some pain, even if only from local anaesthetic injection, and their cooperation obtained to ensure they do not move and injure themselves or the operator. A gentle but firm approach should be adopted. The use of sedation and topical local anaesthetic creams (e.g. EMLA, Ametop) may prove helpful even with less invasive approaches like PICC placement.

Symptom management

Pain at the site of operation

The optimal use of local anaesthesia

This is vital both for the comfort of the patient and to provide a relaxed still cooperative patient for the operator. Inexperienced operators frequently draw up and inject inadequate volumes of local anaesthetic. A large volume of dilute local anaesthetic delivered over a wide area will be far more effective than a small volume of concentrated solution restricted to a small area. Local anaesthesia takes time to develop, so ideally the solution should be injected and time allowed for its effects to work (ideally about 2–5 minutes). The injected solution can be massaged around to aid spread and reduce local swelling. Remember, any injected air or bubbles will degrade the ultrasound image. Warmed solution is less painful on injection and has less gas in solution to appear as the solution is warmed to body temperature.

The initial injection should be a small volume subcutaneously with a small bore orange (25 g) or blue (23 g) needle. Then dependent on the procedure, larger volumes can be infiltrated in a wider area with a longer needle (a 9 cm 22 g cutting point spinal needle is ideal) to avoid multiple skin punctures. Local anaesthetic can be injected through the vascular access needle as it passes through deeper layers, but care needs to be taken to avoid administration into the target vein. Some operators inject the local anaesthetic under ultrasound guidance as the needle and vein puncture sequence progresses, but this leaves little time for the solution to work.

One per cent lignocaine, with or without adrenaline, is an ideal choice for most applications; 2–5 mL would be adequate for a PICC insertion, 10 mL for a non-tunnelled catheter, 30–40 mL for a tunnelled catheter or port insertion, 10–20 mL for removal of tunnelled catheters. The use of longer acting solutions like bupivacaine is favoured by some operators to provide longer post-operative pain relief, but it takes longer to work and is more cardiotoxic if intravascular injection occurs.

Sedation and analgesia

Most CVC procedures can be satisfactorily performed under local anaesthesia alone. Some patients will be in pain from other causes requiring systemic painkillers to lie comfortably. In other cases, intravenous sedation is often necessary to relax the patient and gain their cooperation during the procedure of CVAD insertion.

Sedation has to be administered judiciously to ensure that the patient is not over sedated, which can result in respiratory compromise and other complications.

The patient must be carefully assessed to determine their likely sensitivity to sedation. The very old and sicker patients are likely to be more sensitive. Younger, fitter and very anxious patients are likely to require more sedation. Patients with liver and renal impairment may be more sensitive and may have delayed clearance of drugs. Patients who have been previously exposed to narcotics and benzodiazepines are likely to be tolerant and require greater doses of sedation. Concurrent use of analgesia, especially opiates will require careful titration to prevent over-sedation. The indications and safe use of sedation has been extensively debated particularly in relation to dentistry where useful lessons have been learnt (DOH 2000, Royal College of Anaesthetists 2001, American Dental Association 2005).

Sedation and analgesia must always be titrated according to effect on the individual. The aim should be to remain in verbal contact with the patient at all times. Respiratory rate and SaO_2 levels must be closely monitored. Oxygen should be administered routinely to avoid hypoxemia. The antidotes naloxone (reverses opiates) and flumazenil (reverses benzodiazepines) must be available, but it should be appreciated that their short duration of action may lead to re-sedation after about 20 minutes. Experienced staff must be available to look after and monitor the sedated patient both during and after the procedure, this should not be the operator alone. Patients must not be allowed to drive within 24 hours or go home alone. Occasional adult patients and smaller children will require a general anaesthetic to perform procedures.

Prophylactic antiemetic drugs may be helpful if the patient is suffering from nausea and vomiting due to chemotherapy or underlying disease processes.

Pain elsewhere in the body

Skeletal or other pain from underlying malignancy is very common and such patients may have real difficulty in lying still on their back for the duration of the procedure. Attention to position will help, e.g. with flexion of the hips by putting the legs on pillows in the case of spinal pain. Adequate use of systemic opiates to alleviate pain will be more effective than sedative drugs alone. Success is much more likely if the procedure is performed by a fast, experienced operator to minimise the time they are lying in an uncomfortable position.

Pain and the risk of structural damage during procedures

The use of adequate volumes of local anaesthetic infiltration and judicious use of sedation should allow acceptable conditions in most cases. If the patient still complains of pain, numbness and tingling of the extremities during insertion other factors should be considered. Deeper structures like the vein wall, accompanying arteries and nerves may be sensitive to pressure from the needle, guidewire and larger dilators and such structures are difficult to anaesthetise completely. Some sensation of visceral-type discomfort is normal and the patient should be warned of this. More severe central pain can be a warning sign of blocked vessels, or impending vessel rupture and should alert the operator to stop pushing guidewires or dilators before damage ensues. It may be impossible to safely pass larger stiffer dilators around corners and alternative catheterisation strategies will be required. Deeper injection of local anaesthetic drugs can be performed with or without ultrasound guidance, but a reversible nerve block may occur due to local anaesthetic around the brachial plexus or other nerves in the vicinity of central veins.

The needle may be in contact with the periosteum or nerves supplying the arm, neck or chest. Nerve injury can result with deficits to the upper extremities, diaphragm or hoarseness, but fortunately such damage is rare (see Chapter 12).

Should the patient experience numbness or tingling in the extremities, the operator should immediately withdraw from the affected area and try a slightly different approach. Do not continue to probe in this area and repeatedly reproduce these symptoms. It is likely that the risk of damage is directly related to the number of needle passes and the depth the needle is inserted.

Knowledge about such complications is essential. The routine use of ultrasound should ensure first pass puncture of the anterior vein wall without transfixion, and the shortest route through tissues and no excessive exploration with the needle. Newer high-resolution ultrasound devices are capable of imaging larger nerve bundles, e.g. the brachial plexus allowing avoidance of such structures. Operators should be aware of the ultrasound appearances of nerves (Marhofer *et al.* 2005).

Confused patients

The reason for confusion, as well as the degree of confusion, must be established as this will impact on the procedure. A patient with a head injury may be restless and uncooperative, and it may be unwise to sedate the patient or place in the Trendelenburg position. An elderly confused patient may be reasonably cooperative during the procedure, but eventual displacement of the device will be highly likely.

The patient who cannot be safely sedated at the bedside, and who is uncooperative, is best referred for a procedure under general anaesthesia. If the operator deems that the patient will be sufficiently cooperative to perform the procedure safely at the bedside, then he/she should employ the assistance of someone who is familiar to the patient and who will hopefully be able to encourage cooperation. Issues of patient or third-party consent should be explored as well as the overall risk benefits of the procedure and anaesthesia/sedation.

To reduce the risk of displacement of a tunnelled CVC, the device should be tunnelled out of the patient's view and grasp. This is usually posterior across the shoulder and onto the back. A PICC should be inserted into the dominant arm and kept covered post-insertion. Use of securing devices, e.g. statlocks can make the device more difficult to remove by the restless, confused patient.

Respiratory disease

Most respiratory problems can be anticipated and avoided by thorough preassessment of the patient. Care should be taken to avoid exacerbation of pre-existing conditions that may affect respiratory function, by avoiding prolonged placement in the Trendelenburg position and inadvertent overdose of sedation.

Assessment should include the respiratory rate, ability to talk, oxygen requirements and the presence of cyanosis. Pleural effusions, large abdominal girth and ascites will further interfere with the mechanics of pulmonary physiology if the patient is kept in the Trendelenburg position for a prolonged period (Jubber 2004).

Patients suffering from gastroesophageal reflux disease should be questioned to establish whether they can tolerate lying flat for a prolonged period without adverse effect (Roka 2005). Ideally, they should be kept nil per mouth prior to CVC insertion.

Patients who already have a degree of respiratory compromise, or who after assessment suggest that prolonged placement in the Trendelenburg position will become compromised, should be kept in a semi-recumbent position during preparation for CVC insertion. Once the catheter has been inserted, the patient should again be returned to the semi-recumbent position during suturing and dressing of the device. Throughout the procedure, SaO_2 must be monitored and oxygen administered as necessary. Occasional patients may need general anaesthesia and positive pressure ventilation to tolerate such procedures.

Unexpected and prolonged attempts at cannulation may result in the patient becoming hypoxic, hypercapnic, tachypnoeic or restless. The procedure should be put on hold, oxygen administered and the patient sat up. If the patient recovers, and it seems appropriate to proceed, this should be done with caution and close observation for recurrence of symptoms of respiratory distress.

When considering inserting a CVC into a patient with an existing pneumothorax, large pleural effusion, or pneumonectomy, it is advisable to insert the catheter into the affected side to avoid further respiratory compromise in the case of inadvertent puncture of the pleura on the side of the healthy lung.

Coughing

Some patients will be prone to coughing especially when lying flat, e.g. the patient with a tracheostomy, the patient suffering from gastroesophageal reflux disease, or those in the early stages of treatment for acute lymphoma. Similar considerations about head-down positioning apply, as discussed above.

Prevention of coughing during insertion of a CVC is vital in preventing serious complications to the patient, such as arterial puncture, haemothorax, pneumothorax, air embolism or perforated trachea. The patient must be assessed to ensure that he/she can tolerate lying flat, and that their cough can be suppressed if necessary. Patients with an intractable cough may benefit initially by insertion of a PICC, until the coughing resolves. Intravenous opioids suppress cough reflexes and may be a useful adjunct to sedation.

The patient must be instructed to notify the operator if he/she feels the need to cough, and to suppress this need until the operator instructs the patient that it is safe to do so. Crucial stages during the procedure where coughing would be undesirable include: during needle insertion into the vein and insertion of the introducer and catheter. The procedure may need to be abandoned if coughing is uncontrollable.

Snoring

A patient who is snoring has a partially obstructed airway, which will result in lower intrathoracic pressures on inspiration. This may increase the risk of an air embolus. Deep sedation is usually the cause of snoring. This can be avoided by judicious administration of sedation to meet the patient's individual needs. The head-tilt and chin-lift manoeuvre by a trained assistant, who should be there to monitor the patient anyway, should alleviate the obstruction.

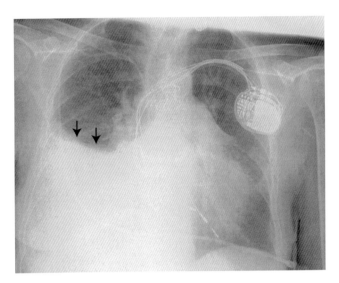

Figure 11.1 A chest X-ray of an elderly lady with significant heart disease making it difficult for her to lie flat. The X-ray shows a chronic right pleural effusion (arrows), the ring of a prosthetic mitral valve replacement and a permanent dual chamber pacing system inserted by the left subclavian route. There are two old disconnected pacing wires left in situ and two attached to the existing box. A Hickman line has been inserted via the right axillary subclavian route.

Cardiovascular disease

The patient who has decompensated heart failure will not tolerate lying flat or the head-down position, similar considerations apply as in respiratory failure as described above. Breathless morbidly obese patients or those with congestive heart failure will generally have high central venous pressures and may not be required to lie flat or head down to cannulate veins; assess venous pressure clinically or with ultrasound first and if suitable perform procedures in sitting or semi-recumbent position (see Figure 3.5).

Pre-existing arrhythmias may indicate that the myocardium could be hypersensitive. The presence of implanted pacemakers or defibrillators and their internal leads should be noted and will also dictate the insertion site, which should be on the contralateral side to the implanted box. Temporary pacing wires are not mechanically fixed to the myocardium, so run the risk of dislodgement during insertion of other vascular access devices. The tips of permanent wires embedded in the myocardium are at low risk of dislodgment (Figure 11.1). Infection of permanent implanted cardiac devices is a real risk from catheter-related sepsis from CVADs, with very serious consequences for the patient as such devices are not easily or safely removed.

Venous stenosis

An accurate CVAD history is important to aid anticipation of venous stenosis. Renal, home total parenteral nutrition, cystic fibrosis and long-term oncology/haematology patients are at particular risk due to insertion of numerous long-term catheters.

If a patient has an extensive history of catheter insertions look for dilated venous collaterals on the chest wall or elsewhere, which should alert the operator to the presence of an underlying venous stenosis (see Chapters 2, 3 and 10). Ultrasound gives further information and should be routinely used to assess patency before starting in such cases. A widely patent vein with respiratory variation in size, appropriate forward Doppler flow and the absence of collateral veins suggests open access to the central veins. If problems have been experienced or anticipated, it is advisable to obtain a venogram prior to attempting a bedside insertion, to ensure patency of the central thoracic veins. Warn the patient beforehand if you anticipate difficulties so there is no embarrassment in having to stop the procedure, nor pressure to proceed at all costs with the risk of complications.

Problems with venous access

There are a number of reasons why the operator may fail to gain access:

(1) *Inability to cannulate the chosen vein*: In many situations, the first choice of site of access would be the right internal jugular vein, and the size and patency of this vessel should be assessed with ultrasound (NICE 2002) (see Chapters 5 and 9). If the chosen vein is unsuitable look elsewhere. Flat, easily compressible veins, with marked collapse on inspiration, indicate that a patient is hypovolaemic and cannulating the vessel may prove to be a challenge. Ensuring the patient is well hydrated and optimally positioned prior to the procedure will aid cannulation. Time the needle puncture of the vein with ultrasound guidance so that the vein is as full as possible by asking the patient to stop breathing or perform a Valsalva manoeuvre. Empty veins will often have to be transfixed with the needle and then access gained as the needle is slowly withdrawn. Sharp fine bore needles and appropriate guidewires (e.g. micropuncture kits) may be helpful in such circumstances.

(2) *Failure to pass the guidewire centrally*: In most cases, guidewires will pass centrally without problems. If screening is not used or unavailable then the presence of ectopic beats is a sign of central passage of guidewires. Patients will complain of pain behind the ear if the guidewire is passed upwards in the neck. Guidewires and catheters can be seen to be misplaced in the neck or contralateral side with ultrasound. In most situations, guidewires can be passed centrally under fluoroscopic guidance without difficulty.

There are multiple reasons why a guidewire will not pass centrally including coiling in the vein, passage into branches of the vein, vein tortuosity, acute angulation of vessels, congenital anatomical variation and vein stenosis (see Chapters 3 and 10). Any resistance to passage should raise suspicion of a problem and if simple repositioning of the needle, guidewire or patient is not successful then further imaging will be required and if unavailable the procedure at that site must be abandoned. If screening is available then fluoroscopy with injection of X-ray contrast through the needle or a short cannula in the vein should allow identification of any abnormal anatomy, even without a formal venogram sequence (Figures 11.2–11.4). Such images can then guide further approaches elsewhere, referrals to more specialist services, or interventions like angioplasty and stenting (Figure 11.5). There

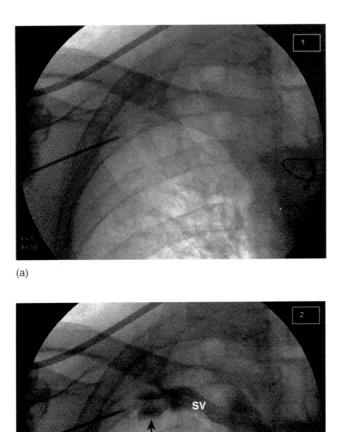

Figure 11.2 (a) A needle has been inserted via the right axillary/subclavian vein with ultrasound guidance. (b) X-ray contrast injected through the needle demonstrates free flow via the subclavian vein (SV) to the superior vena cava (SVC) using limited fluoroscopy without a formal venography sequence. There are sternal wires from previous open heart surgery. (Compare with formal venogram as shown in Figure 7.2). There are paravalvular sinuses outlined (arrow).

are detailed descriptions of such techniques elsewhere (Pieters *et al.* 2003) and in Chapter 10.

(3) *Persistent redirecting Seldinger wire*: This is common after subclavian or left internal jugular access due to the variable angles between major veins; the gentle curves shown in anatomy texts regrettably are not the norm in all cases, particularly the elderly. More seriously, it may be due to a venous stenosis in a patient who has had

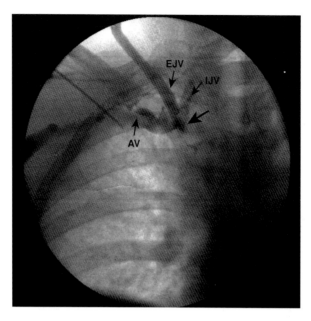

Figure 11.3 An introducing needle has been passed into the right axillary subclavian vein (AV) with ultrasound and blood is freely aspirated but the guidewire will not pass centrally. Injection of contrast through the needle shows free reflux of blood up to the external jugular (EJV), limited flow up to the internal jugular (IJV) and no flow centrally (thick arrow). This is typical of appearances seen with central vein blockage, in this case at the junction of the right innominate and IJV. It is a clear signal to move to another site or seek specialist advice.

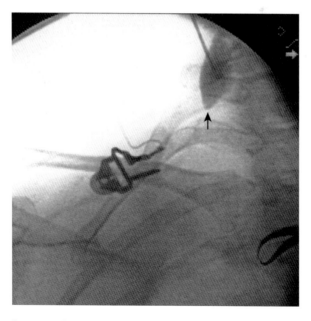

Figure 11.4 An introducing needle has been passed into the right IJ, blood is freely aspirated but a guidewire will not pass. A limited fluoroscopy image demonstrates no central flow of contrast and a typical cone-shaped appearance of a stenosis. This prompts the operator to consider alternative sites.

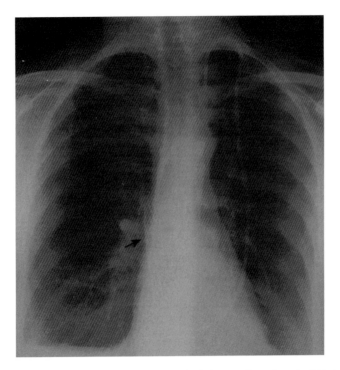

Figure 11.5 Chest X-ray post-Hickman line insertion via the left internal jugular vein. This lady has had a stent (arrow) inserted to open up a narrowed lower SVC following multiple catheters during 18 years of home total parenteral nutrition. The tip of the catheter passes through the stent into the right atrium (RA).

previous central venous catheter insertions, or due to other congenital or acquired venous anomalies.

Measures to overcome this difficulty include positioning of the head or pressure to occlude the internal jugular vein if during the subclavian approach, the guidewire appears to be migrating upwards. A downward direction of the needle will also help to direct the wire down the correct route. Ask the patient to take a deep breath on advancing the wire. Alternatively, use screening with a preshaped cannula to direct the wire centrally. If the wire will not redirect, it is important not to force it. The procedure should be halted, or an alternative access site tried.

(4) *Inability to pass catheters centrally*: Catheters and dilators which pass directly over a guidewire will generally pass centrally without problems, but it should be appreciated that stiffer devices may not be able to follow a guidewire around tight corners with the risk of vein damage if excessive force is used. If passage is not easy then screening should be used to ensure that such guidewires, dilators and catheters are sequentially passing safely into a central intravascular position. Guidewires can also kink and knot (Burns 1989, Carpentier 1991).

There are specific devices (e.g. Braun Certofix) where the guidewire tip, protruding from a central venous catheter, is used as a sensing electrode for the trace on an ECG monitor. As the guidewire and catheter enters the right atrium, a character-istic change in the size of the P wave is seen verifying central placement and the approximate correct length of the catheter. Such devices appear to work best with

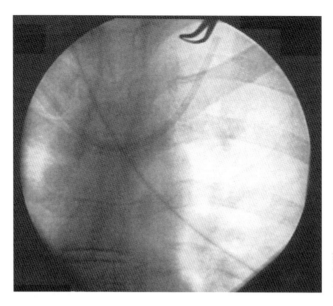

Figure 11.6 Intraoperative screening demonstrates a Hickman catheter has passed from the right subclavian access across into the left innominate vein and upwards into the left internal jugular vein. This is usually easily rectified with guidance from screening.

right-sided catheters but cannot reliably differentiate between venous, arterial or extravascular placement within or adjacent to the heart (Schummer *et al.* 2003, 2004).

Catheters which pass through a cannula or sheath may not pass to a correct position centrally even if the guidewire was correctly sited initially (Figures 11.6–11.8). This is particularly common when soft silicone catheters are passed through an introducer sheath for number of reasons:

(a) Sheaths (particularly larger bore) kink easily on traversing corners. The sheath may need to be withdrawn in order for it to straighten and allow passage of the catheter.

(b) Sheaths can, on occasions, be misplaced outside the vein. The devices may or may not have initially been in the vein (Figure 11.9).

(c) There is not enough torque rigidity in the catheter to allow it to negotiate a correct central passage, even with the aid of screening. If the manoeuvres discussed above do not work then with screening pass a long narrow gauge Teflon-coated guidewire (e.g. Terumo) through the device to increase the rigidity and torque in the catheter. This will usually allow enough control to allow passage centrally. The guidewires in most insertion kits are generally only designed in length and gauge for inserting the dilator and sheath, and will not be long or narrow enough to pass through the catheter for such manoeuvres. Separate guidewires will be required and should be stocked ready for use.

(d) Fine bore thin-walled catheters may be difficult to see on X-rays. If doubt exists as to catheter position, it is advisable to fill the deadspace of the catheter with X-ray contrast to make it more radio-opaque.

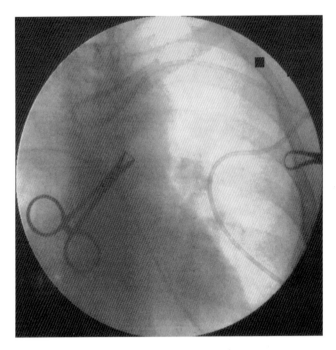

Figure 11.7 A Hickman line has been inserted via the left axillary subclavian vein but does not aspirate blood, intraoperative screening shows the device looped back on itself. This needs to be straightened out with screening control.

   (e) PICCs may be commonly inserted at the bedside without screening. The catheter may be found on chest X-ray immediately following insertion to have fed up into the jugular vein, across into the opposite subclavian or back down an arm vein. In these cases, it is worth leaving the PICC in overnight or flushing fairly forcefully with 20 mL 0.9% saline in a 20 mL syringe and then repeating the X-ray (use of a 20 mL syringe will ensure the pressures are kept low enough to avoid splitting the catheter). This will usually result in the PICC moving into the superior vena cava (Figure 11.10) (Rastogi *et al.* 1998, Banks 1999) and if successful avoids exposing the patient to the risks and discomfort of inserting a new PICC.

Needles

Blockage of the cannulation needle is more likely to occur from clot if the patient has a high platelet count or is receiving a platelet transfusion. Fat of other tissue may also block needles. It is prudent to flush the cannulation needle with normal saline between each cannulation attempt to ensure patency of the needle.

   Needles blunt very quickly if bone is hit or on repeated skin puncture. It may be very difficult to access an empty vein with a blunt needle as excess force on its passage through tissues completely flattens the vein. Do not hesitate to ask for new needle.

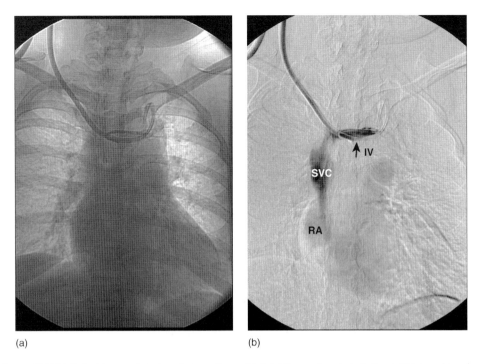

(a)   (b)

Figure 11.8 (a) A dual lumen dialysis catheter with a split distal tip was inserted via the right internal jugular vein. It has passed over the midline to the left and operators are concerned as to its position. (b) X-ray contrast injected with a venogram sequence shows free flow centrally through the right heart and into the pulmonary arteries confirming its position in the left innominate vein. Its position could then be safely corrected with screening.

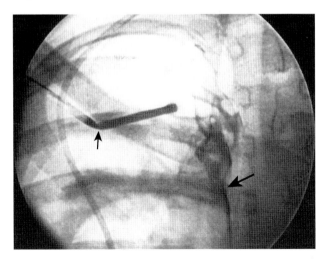

Figure 11.9 A splitting sheath (partially kinked – small arrow) has been inserted via a right subclavian puncture, but the catheter cannot be passed inwards and no blood is flowing out. Contrast injected through the sheath is seen flowing into the right pleural space (large arrow) indicating obvious misplacement and the need to remove the device, bearing in mind it may have traversed the vein first to get to this position. A pneumothorax is likely to follow.

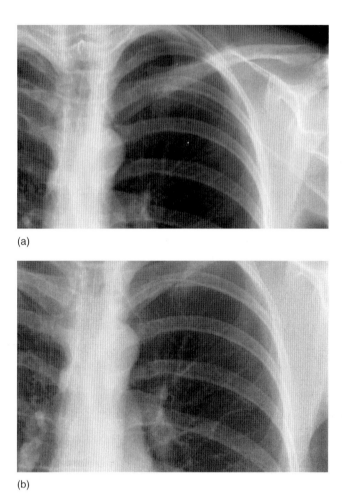

(a)

(b)

Figure 11.10 (a) PICC inserted from the left arm is seen on post-insertion X-ray to be curled back on itself in the left subclavian vein. (b) After flushing, the catheter has straightened out into a satisfactory position. See text for further discussion.

Also, be aware that some manufacturer's kit contains relatively blunt needles from the outset. An initial skin puncture with a scalpel (number 11 is ideal) and blunt dissection with forceps will also help in this situation to minimise the tissues the needle must pass through before hitting the vein.

Arterial puncture

As veins run in close approximation to arteries, inadvertent puncture of an artery during a blind cannulation attempt can be occasionally expected. If unrecognised, arterial catheterisation may occur. The routine use of ultrasound needle guidance should dramatically reduce the risk of these complications (see Chapter 12). On completion of the procedure, the ward staff should be made aware that an artery was punctured, and should be asked to observe the patient for haematoma formation and potential sequelae.

Problems with tunnelling catheters

The tunnelled component of cuffed catheters will occasionally give rise to difficulties if attention to detail is not pursued (Docktor *et al.* 1999). The choice of site for the tunnel tract and exit site should be discussed with the patient, and examination of the chest wall will indicate restrictions to some areas in many patients (see Chapter 3).

Sharp trocars are the easiest to tunnel, but great care is needed in pushing them towards major vessels (e.g. the carotid artery), nerves or the pleura to avoid major visceral damage. Care is also required to avoid injury to operator or assistant. If the safer blunt-ended tunnelling rods are used then the following suggestions may help:

(1) After skin incisions, make a pocket in deeper tissues at both ends of the proposed tunnel tract with blunt dissection with artery forceps. A covering of tissues over the end of the tunnelling rod may need incision with a scalpel before the rod can be pulled free.
(2) Put a 45° curve in the metal tunnelling rod as this will help the rod to exit the tissues at an angle and not pass under the drapes on exit. Soft plastic dilators may be impossible to pass through tough tissues. It is worth stocking some separate metal tunnelling rods for the difficult case.
(3) If tunnelling a longer distance from the chest wall to neck, it may be easier to perform this in two stages with a separate puncture site between the two tracts.
(4) For larger bore catheters, two separate puncture sites in the neck 2–4 cm apart will make the 180° turn gentler and avoid catheter kinking (Figures 11.11 and 11.12).
(5) Do not attempt to take larger bore catheters through a greater than 90° curve, as a kink will occur in the catheter. Instead, create more than one puncture site to create a tissue bridge to graduate the curve.
(6) If the tunnel tract does not closely approximate the tract leading down to the vein then a kink may occur. If this happens and the catheter does not easily 'sink out of view into the tissues' when pushed inwards then the connecting pockets need to be enlarged and deepened by blunt dissection. A similar problem can occur if the tunnel tract is too superficial under the skin. Often a fine bridge of tissue can be seen obstructing the course of the catheter and this can be divided with a fine pair of scissors.
(7) Blunt tunnelling rods do not pass easily through the mobile tissues in the neck. Consider the use of a small mosquito artery forceps to perform the same function more easily.

Port insertion

The site of the port should be dictated by its size and shape and patient needs. For patients with small bore low-profile devices, the upper arm on the non-dominant side

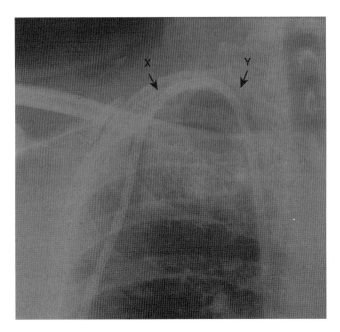

Figure 11.11 A large bore long-term cuffed dialysis catheter inserted via the right internal jugular vein. Two separate puncture holes in the neck (arrows) lessens the acute angles that the catheter has to take at points X and Y ensuring the catheter is not kinked, which would reduce blood flows through it.

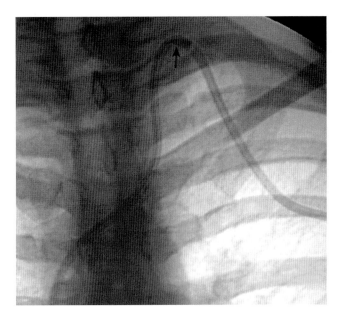

Figure 11.12 A large bore double lumen Hickman catheter has been inserted via the left internal jugular vein. The catheter can be seen to be kinking (arrow) which will reduce flows or cause blockage of the lumen. This can be avoided by ensuring there is adequate tissue bridge as the catheter passes through a 180° turn. This can be achieved by two puncture holes in the neck (Figure 11.11).

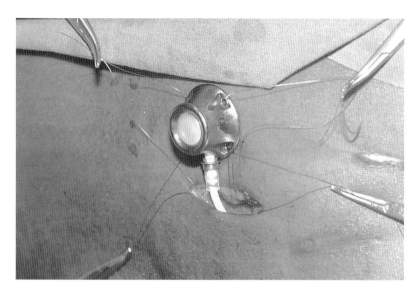

Figure 11.13 A port is being reinserted in this patient for repeated venesection of blood for the treatment of thalassaemia. The port pocket has been prepared and non-absorbable sutures have been inserted and passed through the retaining holes in the base of the device. The port can then be slid into the pocket and the anchoring sutures tied off. This avoids difficulties in trying to insert sutures with a device tightly fitted within the pocket.

may be ideal. Larger ports are best sited over the chest wall, avoiding mobile tissues with the rib cage behind to provide support during needle insertion. The port pocket and incision should be a tight fit around the port to minimise tissue dissection and the potential for haematoma formation. This in turn should reduce the risk of infection or 'capsize' of the port. It is difficult to insert securing the sutures once the port is in its pocket. Therefore, insert the sutures first and then slide the port into its pocket over the sutures and then tie off (Figure 11.13).

Ports sites are painful for the first few days post-insertion. If the port is to be accessed within the first few days, consider leaving an access needle in situ to avoid the need for painful pressure during needle insertion. Mark the site of the membrane with a sterile surgical marker pen to help early access of a swollen site.

Conclusion

Successful safe central venous access requires attention to detail at all stages of the procedure both by the original operator and other staff looking after the patient.

References

American Dental Association (2005). Policy statement: the use of conscious sedation, deep sedation and general anesthesia in dentistry. Available at http://www.adafoundation.org/prof/resources/positions/statements/statements_anesthesia.

Banks N (1999). Positive outcome after looped peripherally inserted central catheter malposition. *Journal of Intravenous Nursing* 22:14–18.

Burns AM, Shelly MP, Abbott TR (1989). Kinking of a Seldinger wire. *Anaesthesia* 44:267.

Carpentier JP, Braz da Silva J, Choukroun G (1991). Formation of a knot in a J spiral metallic guide: a complication of the Seldinger method. *Canadian Anesthesiology* 39:277–278.

Docktor BL, Sadler DJ, Gray RR *et al.* (1999). Radiologic placement of tunnelled central catheters. *American Journal of Roentgenology* 173:457–460.

DOH (Department of Health) (2000). *A Conscious Decision: A Review of the Use of General Anaesthesia and Sedation in Primary Dental Care*. Department of Health, London.

Jubber AS (2004). Respiratory complications of obesity. *International Journal of Clinical Practice* 58:573–580.

Marhofer P, Greher M, Kapral S (2005). Ultrasound guidance in regional anaesthesia. *British Journal of Anaesthesia* 94:7–17.

National Institute for Clinical Excellence (NICE) (2002). *Guidance on The Use of Ultrasound Locating Devices for Placing Central Venous Catheters*. Technology Appraisal Guidance – No. 49. September 2002.

Pieters PC, Tisnado J, Mauro MA (2003). *Venous Catheters: A Practical Manual*. Thieme Medical Publishers, New York.

Rastogi S *et al.* (1998). Spontaneous correction of the malpositioned percutaneous central venous line in infants. *Pediatric Radiology* 28:694–696.

Roka R *et al.* (2005).Prevalence of respiratory symptoms and diseases associated with gastroesophageal reflux disease. *Digestion* 71:92–96.

Royal College of Anaesthetists (2001). *Implementing and Ensuring Safe Sedation Practice for Healthcare Procedures in Adults*. Report of an Intercollegiate Working Party. Available at www.rcoa.ac.uk.

Schummer W *et al.* (2004). Central venous catheters – the inability of 'intra-atrial ECG' to prove adequate positioning. *British Journal of Anaesthesia* 93:193–198.

Schummer W, Herrmann S, Schummer C, *et al.* (2003). Intra-atrial ECG is not a reliable method for positioning left internal jugular vein catheters. *British Journal of Anaesthesia* 91:481–486.

Chapter 12

Complications of central venous access

Andrew R. Bodenham and Liz Simcock

Introduction

The insertion and use of a central venous catheter (CVC) exposes the patient to a wide range of potential complications. At best such complications may bring discomfort and anxiety, or delay the patient's treatment regime. At worst they may lead to life-threatening events such as vessel perforation, sepsis or embolism. It is vital that those who insert CVCs and those responsible for patients' subsequent care are aware of how to prevent and recognise complications, and how to respond appropriately when they occur.

Pneumothorax

Pneumothorax is the presence of air in the pleural space between the lungs and the chest wall. It may be caused when a needle, guidewire, dilator or catheter which is used to access the subclavian or jugular veins inadvertently punctures the lung (Perdue 2001, Weinstein 2001, Dougherty and Lister 2004).

Prevention

The risk of pneumothorax is highest when inexperienced operators use a 'blind' approach to access the vein, and can be reduced with the use of ultrasound (NICE 2002). However, practitioners experienced in using a 'blind' landmark approach can achieve an extremely low rate of pneumothorax, by careful technique (e.g. keeping the needle flat against the skin and not at an angle in the subclavian approach).

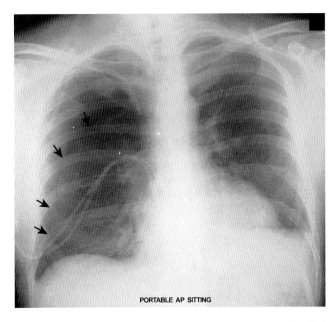

PORTABLE AP SITTING

Figure 12.1 A right pneumothorax following a Hickman line insertion via the right subclavian vein. The lung edge is arrowed. This was recognised when the patient developed respiratory distress 2 hours after the procedure, and was successfully drained.

Recognition

Aspiration of air into the syringe during advancement of the needle should raise suspicion that the lung had been punctured, but pneumothorax may also occur without the operator being aware of a problem during the procedure. Pneumothorax may be clinically silent or may lead to signs and symptoms of varying severity including increased respiratory rate, respiratory distress, cough, tachycardia, chest pain, reduced oxygen saturation levels and hypotension. There are characteristic changes on plain X-rays (Figure 12.1), but these may be subtle in patients with intrinsic lung disease or positive pressure ventilation where the lung does not collapse completely.

Some authors (Drewett 2000a) recommend screening for clinically silent insertion-related pneumothorax by carrying out a delayed chest X-ray a few hours after catheter insertion.

Management

A small, asymptomatic pneumothorax may resolve spontaneously and monitoring of the patient will be all that is required. If the patient is experiencing respiratory distress, supportive care including oxygen therapy should be commenced and vital signs monitored. An urgent medical/surgical assessment should be carried out. In severe cases, aspiration or drainage of the pneumothorax may be necessary, and the patient may require critical care support. Ventilated patients will usually require a chest drain to avoid the development of a so-called tension pneumothorax.

Air embolism

Minor volumes of air embolus (air entering the venous circulation) during fluid infusion and injection of medications is very common and usually causes no harm to the patient, but should be minimised by careful technique. They will distribute in the circulation following the effects of blood flow and gravity. Such bubbles are visible in the jugular veins at open neck surgery in the head-up position. Air bubbles will be trapped in the pulmonary capillaries and get absorbed over time. In contrast, small air bubbles in the arterial circulation may cause major problems if they pass into the brain to cause a transient ischaemic attack (TIA) or stroke. Certain patients may be at particular risk from smaller volume venous air embolism due to air bubbles passing from the venous to the arterial systemic circulation, via right to left heart shunts, e.g. patients with atrial or ventricular septal defects.

Major air embolus is a potentially fatal complication, and most commonly occurs during insertion or removal of the CVC. It is unclear what volume of air represents a significant risk to the patient. During catheter insertion, significant air entry is most likely to happen through a large bore non-valved open introducer sheath in the time between withdrawal of the dilator and insertion of the catheter (Vesely 2001). During catheter removal, air embolus may occur as the catheter is being withdrawn from the vein (Drewett 2000b), or via the track left by the catheter after removal (McCarthy 1995). With tunnelled catheter removal, there is the added risk that the catheter may accidentally be snapped or severed in the attempt to dissect the cuff within the tunnel, thus allowing air to enter the vein, unless the internal tip of the catheter is valved.

The risk of air embolism is increased if there is a sudden reduction in venous pressure, if, for example, the patient takes a sharp breath in, coughs or snores suddenly. The chances of a serious air embolism during the insertion or removal of PICCs is probably far less than with centrally inserted catheters due to the position of the entry site and the relatively small size of the vein and the catheter. Chronic low-grade air embolism due to small leaks in CVCs has also been described causing pulmonary oedema (Fitchet and Fitzpatrick 1998).

Prevention during catheter insertion

Good technique and careful patient assessment are crucial in preventing air embolism. If the patient is dehydrated, unable to lie flat or has an uncontrolled cough, the risk is increased (Drewett 2000). The operator should assess for these risks prior to the procedure, possibly considering an alternative approach (e.g. a PICC) as a short-term solution until clinical symptoms resolve.

Various measures can increase the pressure in the vein at crucial points during the insertion of the catheter and therefore reduce the risk of air embolism. These include ensuring the patient is well hydrated and positioned so that the relevant vein is below the level of the heart. For upper body CVCs, this means tipping the bed head down, in the Trendelenburg position. For femoral catheters, the head of the bed should be tilted up. For PICCs, the patients' arm should be positioned below heart level. Minimising the time between removal of the dilator from a sheath and insertion of the catheter will also reduce the risk of air entering the vascular system.

In upper body catheter placement, this part of the procedure should never be carried out while the patient is coughing or during inspiration as the changes in vascular pressure may result in air being sucked in via the introducer. The operator may time this part of the procedure to coincide with the patient's expiration. If the patient is awake, they may be instructed to hold their breath or perform the Valsalva manoeuvre. The Valsalva manoeuvre is thought to be effective in reducing the risk of air embolism (Wysoki 2001), but requires a cooperative patient and good communication. Some patients when asked to 'hold their breath' may interpret this as meaning that they should take a large breath which would actually increase the risk of embolism. If deep sedation is used, there is a risk that the patient may suddenly snore, increasing the risk of air entry. Other techniques useful in reducing the risk of air embolism during catheter insertion include pinching the sheath and using a valved system. Similar principles apply during catheter removal (see Chapter 14).

Recognition

Air entering the venous system via an introducer during catheter insertion may be audible to the operator; this sound has been described by one operator as 'a worrying gurgle'. Another called it 'a whooshing sound'. On the other hand, air embolism can occur without the operator being aware that anything untoward has occurred. Careful monitoring of the patient's oxygen saturation levels and vital signs during CVC insertion should be standard. Air embolism may be clinically silent or may be accompanied by any or all of the following: anxiety, cyanosis, dyspnoea, tachycardia, hypotension, chest pain, loss of consciousness, cardiorespiratory arrest and death. Air bubbles in the circulation have characteristic ultrasound appearances and echocardiography provides definitive evidence of air in the cardiac chambers.

Management

Air embolism is an emergency situation, as larger volumes will cause cardiorespiratory arrest. The portal for further air entry must be closed by digital pressure, occlusive dressings or other manoeuvres. The patient position should be changed so that the area of air entry is below the heart (head down tilt for upper body access sites). Careful monitoring and 100% oxygen therapy should be commenced if air embolism is suspected, and if symptomatic the patient will require immediate supportive care. It is customary to turn the patient onto their left side and positioned with the head lower than the body to encourage the air embolus to move to the right atrium preventing it from obstructing blood flow to the right ventricle and lungs (Belcaster 1997). The effectiveness of this manoeuvre is questioned by Vesely (2001) who suggests that it may be ineffective or even detrimental.

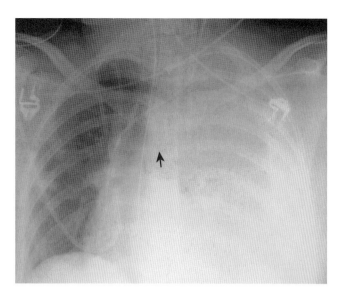

Figure 12.2 A 12-fr introducer sheath for a pulmonary artery catheter has been inserted via the left internal jugular route but has not traversed the corner and has entered the left pleural space (arrow marks its tip). Compare the correct course of the multilumen catheter passing into the SVC also from the left internal jugular vein. Bleeding around the catheter is producing an enlarging left haemothorax with mediastinal shift. A right internal jugular Hickman catheter and nasogastric tube and endotracheal tube are also present. The misplaced catheter was left in place to prevent massive bleeding whilst preparations were made to perform a thoracotomy to repair the vein damage.

If a catheter is already present in the right atrium, it may be possible to aspirate air. Vesely (2001) cites isolated cases where this has been successful but warns that given the low likelihood of success, insertion of a right atrial catheter specifically for this purpose is probably not justified.

Pleural effusions

This occurs as a result of blood, infused fluids, lymph fluid or a mixture of fluids leaking into the low-pressure pleural space. Bleeding may occur due to great vessel damage as the major arteries and veins are in proximity to the pleural space (see below) (Figure 12.2). Infused fluids, e.g. crystalloids, colloids, intravenous feeds and blood products have all on occasions been infused into the pleural space when a catheter has not been recognised to have been inserted into the pleural space, or has eroded through the superior vena cava (SVC) wall to lie in the pleural space (Figures 12.3a and 12.3b). Confusion may arise when blood is taken for analysis from the 'central line' which is actually sampling a pleural collection where blood does not always clot fully. Damage to the major lymphatic trunks may result in a lymphatic leak to produce a milky white effusion, a so-called chylothorax.

The patient develops cyanosis, dyspnoea, tachycardia, hypotension and chest pain. Significant symptomatic pleural collections require urgent insertion of a chest drain and

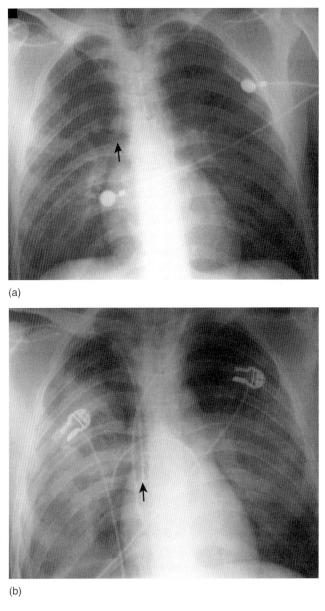

(a)

(b)

Figure 12.3 (a) A right subclavian catheter has been inserted in the accident and emergency department in patient with meningococcal sepsis to monitor the CVP. The initial post-insertion chest X-ray looks satisfactory (arrow marks tip). (b) A second later chest X-ray following further catheter insertions (right internal jugular triple lumen, arrow, and pulmonary artery catheter), and removal of the first catheter shows a right pleural effusion which on drainage is obviously infused fluids from the first catheter. In retrospect, the two central catheter positions are not obviously different due to the proximity of the pleural space and the SVC.

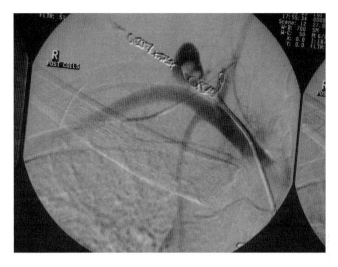

Figure 12.4 A pulsatile swelling was noticed at the base of the right neck following multiple attempts at right internal jugular puncture without ultrasound guidance. Angiography showed a false aneurysm of a branch of the thyrocervical trunk (a branch of the subclavian artery). This image shows the contrast filled aneurysm successfully isolated radiologically by insertion of multiple coils proximally and distally.

referral for specialist advice and interventions. A chest drain is required to remove the fluid, and consideration should then be given to removing the offending CVC which may have eroded a major vessel, so may need surgical or radiology input to close the tear in the vein. Similar problems can occur due to arterial damage in the great vessels and urgent radiology or surgical input is almost always required.

Arterial puncture/catheterisation

Since most of the veins commonly used for central venous catheterisation are situated near major arteries, accidental puncture and indeed catheterisation of an artery rather than a vein is an ever-present hazard. Major arteries commonly at risk include the carotid, vertebral, femoral, subclavian and brachial arteries (see Figure 6.5). Smaller branches of these major vessels may also be damaged (see Figure 12.4).

Well-recognised consequences of arterial damage include haematoma, CVA, false aneurysm, dissection, thrombosis, haemothorax, pericardial tamponade, AV fistula, retroperitoneal haemorrhage and ischaemic limbs. The consequences in part depend on the anatomical location, and further specific details are given in the individual chapters on different routes of access.

Prevention

The extent of the damage caused by accidental arterial puncture can be reduced by ensuring the patient has adequate coagulation status prior to commencing the procedure.

For further discussion refer to Chapter 3. Clearly, in the emergency situation, these precautions may not always be achievable and the risks of inserting a CVAD when coagulation is deranged will need to be weighed against other clinical factors. PICC placement may be safe in the presence of coagulation abnormalities because of the relative ease with which vessels in the arm can be compressed.

The risk of arterial puncture can be almost completely eliminated by the routine use of ultrasound needle guidance. With this technique, the artery and vein are clearly distinguishable and a skilful operator will identify the exact position of both and be able to accurately guide the needle into the vein. When a 'blind' approach is used, the inserter will rely on palpation and their knowledge of anatomy to avoid arterial puncture. Whichever technique is used, however, the risk of arterial puncture remains and the operator must remain alert to any signs that it has occurred. A small bore 'seeker' needle 21 g (green) or 23 g (blue) can also be used to find the vein prior to puncture with the larger introducer needle. Arterial puncture with such fine bore needles is generally safe, but there have been recorded instances of a CVA after insertion of such needles into the carotid (Reuber *et al.* 2002).

Recognition

Accidental arterial puncture with the introducer needle is usually immediately apparent to the operator, with bright red blood back flowing into the needle or syringe in a high-pressure, pulsating flow. However, these signs are not always present (Parikh and Narayanan 2004) and so accidental arterial catheterisation remains a potential hazard.

Various techniques may help to confirm or exclude accidental arterial catheterisation. If the patient's arterial pressure is normal, a standard infusion set with a bag of saline set to a height of less than a metre will show retrograde pulsatile back bleeding if connected to an arterial catheter. Similar observations will follow connection to a CVP manometer set. However, this sign may be absent if the blood pressure is very low. Infusion pump devices will generally alarm and not function. Other useful tests include blood gas monitoring (to show arterial as opposed to venous oxygen saturations), fluoroscopy with dye injection and the use of an electronic pressure transducer (set to arterial pressure range rather than CVP) to show arterial pressure and its characteristic waveform.

It is important to remember that imaging during or after CVAD insertion will not always reveal the presence of the catheter in the arterial system, and clinicians should be aware of the limitations of such imaging. The anatomical proximity of major arteries and veins in the neck and chest may cause difficulties in interpretation, and it is not possible to reliably state whether a catheter is in an artery or a vein in the chest from a plain chest X-ray, hence the often-guarded statements in radiology reports. Such confusion may occur in the presence of normal or abnormal arterial anatomy, as the ascending aorta is adjacent to the SVC (Figures 12.5a, 12.5b and 12.6). In a case described by Parikh and Narayanan (2004), arterial placement of a PICC remained unnoticed for 2 weeks and was recognised only when the patient suffered a stroke as a result of the misplaced catheter. Ricci (1999) cites a case where a catheter was inadvertently introduced via the right common carotid artery into a right-sided aortic arch.

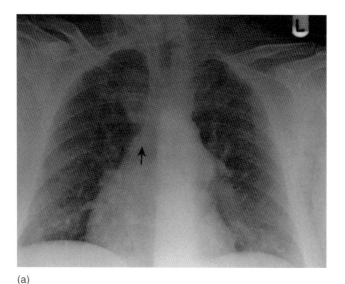

(a)

(b)

Figure 12.5 (a) A central 'venous' catheter passed via the right carotid artery went unrecognised in the ascending aorta on this rather rotated plain chest X-ray, with a perceived position within the SVC (tip shown with arrow). It was recognised after a transient stroke. Other clinical techniques are required to differentiate arterial from venous catheter placement (see text). (b) Axial CT image of same patient showing misplaced catheter crossing the aortic arch into the ascending aorta. P, pleura; C, catheter; SVC, superior vena cava; AA, arch of aorta; T, trachea.

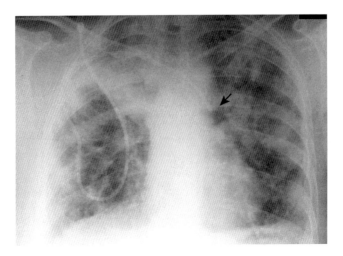

Figure 12.6 A Hickman catheter has been inadvertently passed into the right subclavian artery. This was not recognised by an inexperienced operator at the time of insertion. The post-procedure X-ray alerted staff to the problem as the catheter is seen crossing the midline to lie in the descending aorta (arrow). Contrast with Figure 12.5a.

Management

As soon as accidental arterial puncture is suspected, the needle should be withdrawn from the artery and pressure applied for at least 3–5 minutes. In most cases, this will suffice to prevent any serious sequelae, but it is worth noting that late complications can result from arterial puncture. Mercer-Jones *et al.* (1995) cite one case in which the patient appeared to be stable following arterial puncture but suffered a fatal haemorrhage the following day. Large haematomas require surgical review, and if large require early evacuation to prevent local tissue damage and necrosis. Some develop into a so-called false aneurysm (detectable with Doppler ultrasound) where pulsatile blood flow in and out of the aneurysm is present. The aneurysm is temporarily contained by surrounding tissues. These require surgical or radiological repair (see Figure 12.4).

Inadvertent arterial puncture of the subclavian arteries, innominate arteries and aorta or their branches is dangerous as high pressures mean bleeding does not easily stop, and external pressure cannot be applied. The subclavian arteries bulge into the pleural space on both sides of the chest with the resultant risk of haemothorax after puncture. All carry a significant risk of haemothorax due to bleeding into the low-pressure pleural space. The pericardial reflection ascends up the aortic arch onto its major branches with the result that subclavian artery, innominate artery or aortic damage can cause pericardial tamponade (see below) (Horowitz *et al.* 1991). Similar bleeding can occur from the femoral/iliac arteries into the peritoneal cavity. Similar considerations arise with major venous bleeding (see below).

AV fistula can occur during central venous catheterisation (Zsolt *et al.* 2002) and is thought to be due to simultaneous puncture of both vessel walls during needle insertion. The arterial flow into the low-pressure venous system maintains the defect which over time enlarges and becomes permanent. Fistulas can occur between femoral, subclavian, vertebral (see Figure 5.9), carotid and jugular vessels as well as multiple other sites and typically present late with bruits and signs of venous congestion.

If a larger bore catheter has been inserted into the artery then consideration should be given to the need for surgical removal in theatre or radiological closure with a stent. Optimal management depends on the puncture site, size of catheter, coagulation status, local expertise and other patient factors. Seek senior advice from vascular surgery or radiology. It is unsafe, for example, to provide long-term compression on the carotid in the case of large bore puncture.

Great vein perforation

Perforation of great veins (and arteries) can occur during catheter insertion or at a later time and carries a high risk of morbidity or mortality. The reported incidence varies (Merry *et al.* 1999) and according to Russell and Greiff (2003) 'fatal cardiac or vascular perforation, although fortunately not common, is certainly not rare'. During insertion, perforation is typically associated with direct damage by the needle, guidewire, dilator and introducer (Robinson *et al.* 1995). Perforation occurring later may be related to positioning of the catheter against the vessel wall leading to mechanical and/or chemical damage (Caruso *et al.* 2003). While most reported cases involve the mediastinal vessels, this complication can also arise in patients with catheters sited via the femoral route into the iliac veins or inferior vena cava (IVC) (Nowicka *et al.* 2004).

Tears of large veins may have no sequelae if the vein is surrounded by intact tissues and coagulation is normal, limited bleeding will occur and the pressure from clot will control the haemorrhage. Similar effects may also occur with a smaller puncture to major arteries, but this is far less certain and ongoing bleeding may produce severe local pressure effects (see above, and in respective chapters on each route of access). The major early risk of haemorrhage from great veins or arteries is uncontrolled bleeding into low-pressure spaces in the chest or abdomen. This includes the pleural (see Figure 12.2), pericardial and peritoneal spaces. If unrecognised, this may lead to rapid or delayed collapse and cardiac arrest.

Prevention

Various strategies have been suggested for minimising the risk of this complication. These can be divided as those occurring during insertion procedures and those occurring later when an indwelling catheter perforates the vessel wall.

During insertion, Russell and Greiff (2003) highlight the importance of avoiding overlong dilators and sheaths during insertion of the catheter. The use of soft flexible guidewires and small bore dilators, sheaths and catheters under careful X-ray imaging control will reduce the risk of vessel damage. The routine use of ultrasound to guide vein puncture and adequate operator experience are also vital. Experienced operators will avoid the use of excessive force with dilators, and an awake patient will generally complain of increasing visceral-type pain if excessive force is used, beware of ignoring this sign.

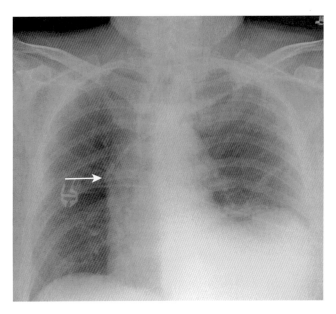

Figure 12.7 The tip of this large bore stiff dialysis catheter (arrow marks its tip) is abutting the wall of the SVC at an acute angle with the risk of pain, thrombosis and erosion into the right pleural space, if left in situ longer term.

Following insertion, Nowicka *et al.* (2004) stress the risks of rigid non-compliant catheters, implying that catheters made of smaller bore more flexible materials may reduce the incidence of perforation. The design of the catheter may also be a factor; the use of catheters with curled 'pigtail' tips, for example, may reduce the risk (Merry *et al.* 1999). Tip position is clearly important in preventing perforation from occurring once the catheter is in situ (Figure 12.7). Reported cases of fatal tamponade in adults and neonates with catheters tips placed in the right atrium have led some to conclude that the tip of the catheter should never be placed within the heart (Wariyar and Hallworth 2001), while others argue that careful atrial tip placement is safe (Cartwright 2002) as long as the tip is placed centrally within the chamber and not abutting the vessel wall. Proponents of vena cava placement tend to favour placing the tip in the lower SVC, but others (Caruso *et al.* 2003) pose the argument that placing the tip in the mid SVC is necessary to ensure the catheter is outside the pericardial reflection to eliminate the risk of cardiac perforation and tamponade. The carina on chest X-ray is a practical marker for the position of the pericardial reflection. However, higher placement in the SVC may increase the risk of damage and thrombosis in the SVC, particularly in catheters placed from the left side. The junction between the left innominate vein and SVC is lower than on the right meaning that there is only short distance between this junction and the pericardial reflection.

Recognition and management

If it is unclear from plain X-rays where the distal section of the catheter lies, this may be verified by further imaging, either injection of contrast or CT (Figures 12.8a

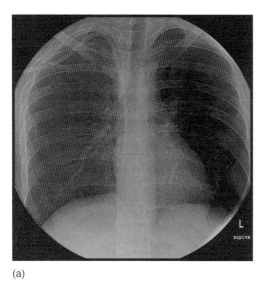
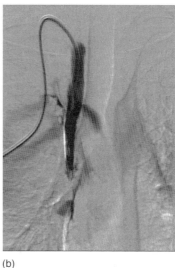

(a)   (b)

Figure 12.8 (a) CVC has passed into the chest but no blood could be aspirated. The position of the catheter initially looked satisfactory on plain X-ray. (b) X-ray contrast injection revealed mediastinal placement. Further contrast injection (not shown) during withdrawal of the catheter verified that no great vessels had been perforated and traversed during the insertion procedure.

and 12.8b). This is particularly true if intra-arterial, pericardial or other visceral placement is suspected, as in the short term it may be safer to leave the device in situ to prevent major haemorrhage or other complications. An informed decision about removal can then be made after consultation with vascular surgeons and radiologists or other specialists.

Perforation of the vena cava is likely to lead to a right haemothorax from bleeding, or an effusion from infused fluids, or a collection of fluid in the mediastinum. Do not automatically remove the catheter as it may be partially blocking the hole in the great vein and slowing bleeding (see Figure 12.2).

Perforation of the lower SVC or right atrium may be a catastrophic event due to the development of pericardial tamponade due to infusion of fluids under pressure or bleeding. Signs include hypotension, muffled heart sounds, high jugular venous pressure, collapse and cardiac arrest. There is a very high mortality, and many cited cases are recognised only at post-mortem (Orme 2007). Immediate supportive care and urgent cardiology or cardiothoracic surgical referral are essential. The diagnosis is confirmed with echocardiography. In the case of pericardial tamponade from infused fluids, it may be possible to aspirate fluid from the pericardium via the catheter to provide short-term relief. Otherwise percutaneous drainage followed by open surgical drainage and repair are generally required.

Damage to other neighbouring structures

Any nearby structure is potentially at risk from needle puncture or other damage. There are reports of damage to the trachea, oesophagus and placement within the cerebrospinal fluid. Fuller listings of complications are available in other detailed texts (Latto 2000) and multiple case reports in the literature.

Lymphatic damage

Larger lymphatic channels follow the course of veins, so unnoticed subclinical damage during attempted vein catheterisation is probably common. Cases of 'lymphatic leak' are reported by Lemmer *et al.* (1987) and by Barnacle and Kleidon (2005), who suggest that puncture of lymphatics is only rarely symptomatic. If significant lymphatic fluid leaks into the pleural space, it presents as an effusion (chylothorax). Thrombosis of the subclavian vein causing blockage to the drainage of the thoracic duct, which carries the majority of the body's lymph fluid, has also been implicated in such effusions (Mallick and Bodenham 2003) (see also Chapter 7).

Nerve damage

Major nerves run parallel to veins in the neurovascular bundles, hence damage is well recognised but fortunately rare. It is well documented in PICCs where the proximity of the brachial veins and nerve can lead to nerve damage (Alomari and Falk 2006). Jugular or subclavian catheters have been known to be associated with damage to the phrenic nerve (Aggarwal 2000), vagus nerve, sympathetic chain and brachial plexus. Ultrasound guidance to ensure first pass vein puncture and visualise larger nerve trunks should minimise such complications.

Cardiac arrhythmias

Definition and incidence

Insertion-related arrhythmias are usually caused by direct stimulation of the myocardium and are a routine occurrence during CVC placement whenever a guidewire or catheter is inserted into the heart (Flaccadori *et al.* 1996). A study by Stuart *et al.* (1992) showed an incidence of 41% for atrial and 25% for ventricular arrhythmias. According to Vesely (2003), 'there is minimal evidence to suggest that this is a significant clinical problem', but there are incidences in the literature of arrhythmias requiring drug therapy or cardioversion (Brothers *et al.* 1988).

Arrhythmias may also occur at a later time once the catheter is in situ, and this phenomenon is seen predominantly with PICCs (Bivins and Callahan 2000), presumably because of the way they move within the venous system following insertion. The distal tip of a PICC has been shown to move up to 9.5 cm when the patient changes the position of their arm, and so even when the tip has been placed outside the atrium, the catheter may still move into the heart and cause arrhythmias. Other types of CVC are less mobile within the body and the tendency is for the catheter to move away from the heart following insertion, as the patient sits up and gravity causes the mediastinal contents to move downwards in relation to the catheter (Vesely 2003). A deep inspiration produces similar effects.

Prevention

During assessment of the patient for CVAD insertion, it is prudent to take note of any cardiovascular history, in particular any existing cardiac arrhythmias. Acute or chronic atrial fibrillation, supraventricular or ventricular ectopic beats may indicate that the myocardium could be hypersensitive. It is also necessary to be aware of any cardiac devices such as pacemakers and implantable defibrillators. This will not only make the operator more aware of an increased risk of arrhythmias, but will also aid selection of the insertion site, which should be on the contralateral side to the insertion site of implanted device.

Other sensible precautions include ensuring that the patient's electrolytes, especially potassium, are corrected prior to insertion so as to be within the acceptable range of normal.

During insertion techniques, the patient's cardiac rate and rhythm must be closely monitored, particularly when advancing the guidewire. The routine use of guidewires with depth markers and an appreciation of the average insertion depth for catheters at each site can significantly reduce the risk of guidewire-related arrhythmias by avoiding insertion of the guidewire into the heart (Stuart *et al.* 1992, Quiney 1994, Lee *et al.* 1996). Others may argue that since most arrhythmias are known to resolve spontaneously after removal of the guidewire, this adjustment in technique is unnecessary. Some operators routinely pass wires with X-ray screening across the right atrium into the IVC to stabilise the wire and confirm venous placement (see Chapter 10).

In the debate concerning CVC tip position, the avoidance of arrhythmias is cited as one argument for placing the tip in the SVC rather than within the right atrium, but there may be other factors to consider. Vesely (2003) discusses this in depth citing various studies showing that in haemodialysis patients the benefits of right atrial placement (improved catheter longevity and function) may outweigh such risks.

The prevention of arrhythmias is more problematic with PICCs, because of the mobility of the catheter once in situ. If the tip of the PICC were to be placed far enough outside the heart to guarantee it did not enter it during arm movements, this might in many patients mean placing it in the upper part of or even outside the SVC, leading to an increased risk of migration and thrombosis. Expert opinion favours lower SVC tip placement (Fletcher 2000), and so the risk of arrhythmias remains.

Recognition and management

Cardiac monitoring during CVC insertion will reveal any arrhythmias and these will usually resolve spontaneously. Should the arrhythmia persist, however, the procedure should usually be halted and assistance obtained to control the cardiac rhythm.

If a patient experiences arrhythmias in the period following insertion, the catheter tip position should be reviewed and the patient should be urgently assessed by the cardiology team including 12-lead ECG. The exception to this may be in the case of a patient who develops palpitations following non-screened PICC insertion and where symptoms resolve immediately upon withdrawal of the PICC by 2 or 3 cm.

Catheter-related sepsis

Infection is the major long-term risk with CVCs. Aspects of infection related to pathogenesis and prevention are extensively covered in Chapter 13 which addresses infection and are not covered here. An overview of other aspects is given.

Choice of catheter

The EPIC guidelines on the prevention of infection in CVCs stress the importance of using the minimum number of lumens consistent with clinical need, since multiple lumens offer multiple opportunities for colonisation (Pratt *et al.* 2007). The guidelines suggest there may also be a role for antimicrobial impregnated catheters in preventing Catheter-related blood stream infection (CRBSI) for patients at high risk requiring short-term central access, but find no justification for the routine replacement of non-tunnelled CVCs over a guidewire as a method of preventing catheter-related infection.

Insertion

Routine antibiotic prophylaxis prior to insertion is not supported by research and may encourage resistant organisms (Pratt *et al.* 2007). During the insertion procedure, the importance of using 'maximal sterile barriers' including sterile gloves, gown and large drapes is paramount, with alcoholic chlorhexidine gluconate 2% as the antiseptic of choice for skin preparation. Following insertion, the CVC should be fixed firmly to the skin, since movement of the catheter in and out of the exit site increases the risk of catheter-related sepsis (Haller and Rush 1992).

Recognition and management

The diagnosis of CVC-related BSI is a complex issue with many questions yet unanswered (Ross 2003). The presence of pyrexia and/or rigor (especially following flushing of the line) in the absence of any other source of infection should raise the suspicion of CVC-related BSI. There may or may not be signs of exit site infection (Safdar and Maki 2002). In the face of clinical signs, blood cultures should be drawn from the catheter as well as peripherally. All lumens should be sampled to avoid false negatives (Robinson 2002, Dobbins *et al.* 2003). Coagulase negative staphylococci are the most common bacteria associated with CVC-related BSI.

The potential seriousness of CVC-related BSI has meant that in many settings removal of the catheter is the standard treatment. This approach has drawbacks. Firstly, it will usually lead to a number of devices being removed unnecessarily. It is well documented that a large proportion of catheters removed because they are suspected of causing BSI are likely to prove sterile in the laboratory (Tighe *et al.* 1996, Kite *et al.* 1997, Hall and Farr 2004). Secondly, experience with long-term CVCs has shown that a certain proportion of infections can be successfully treated (Hall and Farr 2004). Consequently, there is a great clinical need for techniques which can differentiate CVC-related from non-CVC-related BSI, without removal of the catheter, and for guidance as to which infections are likely to be successfully treated and which are not. This is particularly the case for patients who have an ongoing need for reliable central venous access.

Blood cultures taken peripherally and from the CVC of a patient with systemic sepsis are both likely to be positive, and this in itself is not an indication that the catheter is the cause of the infection. Some studies have suggested that quantitative comparison of central and peripheral blood cultures can accurately differentiate catheter-related from non-catheter-related infections. The catheter is considered to be implicated if blood cultures taken centrally exhibit a colony count five times higher than paired peripheral samples, or if they show growth at least 2 hours prior to their peripheral counterpart (Hall and Farr 2004). Analysing blood samples in this way, however, is labour-intensive and costly. Introduction of such techniques as a routine may require research which can demonstrate its cost-effectiveness. Another technique to detect catheter colonisation without removing the line has been developed using a dedicated 'endoluminal brush' which is introduced into the catheter and drawn back along its full length. The bristles are designed to gather any pathogens present on the inside of the catheter and the brush is then sent to the laboratory for analysis. There is evidence to suggest that the accuracy of this method is comparable to established methods of culturing catheters in the laboratory (Tighe *et al.* 1996, Kite *et al.* 1997), although with the obvious advantage that the catheter need not be removed. One drawback is that endoluminal brushing requires specialist skills and equipment and a precise knowledge of the length of the catheter; failure to insert the brush the whole length of the catheter, or inserting it too far so that it enters the blood stream will reduce the accuracy of the test. Concerns have also been raised that endoluminal brushing in itself may carry a risk of embolisation and bacteraemia (Blot *et al.* 2000), although the author has not been able to find published evidence that this is the case.

The wisdom of trying to treat proven CRBSI without removing the catheter will depend on the patient's clinical status, the type of catheter and the causative pathogen. In infected, short-term centrally inserted devices, removal is usually indicated, but in tunnelled and implanted catheters there is more data to support catheter salvage, with published success rates for bacterial infections varying from 18 to 100%. There is some evidence that the use of a heparin and antibiotic lock together with systemic antibiotics may improve the outcome (Krzywda 2002, Hall and Farr 2004). Fungal infections, however, appear to have far less chance of successful treatment and in such cases the catheter should usually be removed (Hall and Farr 2004). The success of treating PICC-related blood stream infections does not appear to have been studied but the author's subjective assessment is that it is as likely to be successful as for tunnelled devices.

Infection at the exit site/tunnel/port pocket

Infection at the exit site, tunnel or pocket should be suspected if there is local erythema and inflammation. There may be accompanying oedema, pain and purulent discharge and pyrexia. Positive wound cultures will aid diagnosis and treatment decisions.

In tunnelled catheters and PICCs, many exit site infections will resolve with antibiotic therapy and daily dressing changes, but infections involving the tunnel or port pocket are notoriously unresponsive to treatment and here catheter removal is indicated (Krzywda 2002).

Attempts to treat exit site infections in non-tunnelled centrally inserted catheters should be informed by the fact that here there is a high risk of subsequent CRBSI as pathogens can migrate easily along the catheter track (Hall and Farr 2004).

Catheter-related vein thrombosis

This section discusses thrombosis formation within a blood vessel around the catheter. Fibrin sheaths and intraluminal clots are dealt with separately in 'patency impairment' below. The insertion and presence of a CVC can result in damage to the vessel wall and lead to thrombosis formation, this being the body's natural response to vascular injury. A variety of intrinsic factors are thought to increase the risk of thrombosis in patients with CVCs. These include recent surgery, a diagnosis of cancer, thrombophilia, chemotherapy, hormonal agents, immobilisation, haemodialysis, pregnancy and diabetes. In addition, the choice of vein, tip position and infection are all thought to influence the risk (Hadaway 1998, Grove and Pevec 2000, Lee and Levine 2000, Marinella *et al.* 2000). Choosing the smallest catheter diameter appropriate to clinical requirements would also seem to be logical.

In the longer–term, thrombus may organise into a fibrin sleeve to give further problems with patency (see Chapter 14).

Recognition

Many thromboses are clinically silent but in those that are not, oedema and pain are the most common clinical signs (Marinella *et al.* 2000). Distension of peripheral or neck veins, erythema, tingling or numbness have also been reported (Cornock 1996, Kayley 1997). In the case of PICCs or subclavian catheters, thrombosis may be suspected when the arm or the hand swells. Unilateral jugular vein thrombosis is typically clinically silent unless infection is also present.

The reported incidence of CVC-related thrombosis varies widely, probably because of variations in definitions, diagnostic methods, patient populations and catheter types (Lee and Levine 2000). The true incidence is thought to be much higher than clinical symptoms would suggest as a large proportion of patients with CVCs have clinically silent thromboses. Balestreri *et al.* (1995) studied 57 oncology patients with CVCs, none of whom had symptoms of thrombosis. Venography revealed the presence of partial or complete thrombosis in 56% of these patients. In a similar study, Allen *et al.* (2000) found a 38% incidence of venous thrombosis in haemodialysis patients with PICCs.

Thrombus formation can occur at any time following insertion of the CVAD. It may initially present as persistent withdrawal occlusion (PWO) or an inability or resistance to flushing. The thrombus probably originates at the point where the device enters the vein, or where there is slight intraluminal damage, e.g. where the device irritates the internal lumen of the vein. The thrombus may enlarge and/or migrate along the length of the device and eventually occlude the tip and the vessels at the point of insertion and more proximally. Pulmonary embolus can be a serious complication following thrombus formation and can occur in up to 12% of catheter-related subclavian or axillary vein thrombosis (Reed and Houng 1999). Patients who develop catheter-related thrombosis are also at increased risk of infection (Marinella *et al.* 2000).

A variety of strategies can be used to minimise the risk of catheter-related vein thrombosis.

The importance of tip position

An increased rate of thrombosis has been demonstrated in suboptimal catheter tip positions. Correct positioning of the tip of the catheter in either the SVC, the IVC or the right atrium is probably the most important strategy for prevention of thrombosis in patients with CVCs (Racadio *et al.* 2001). This will allow the catheter tip to float freely within the blood stream parallel to the vein wall. It is worth quoting from the National Association of Vascular Access Networks (NAVAN) position paper on this subject:

> *When the catheter tip lies outside the SVC, vein curvatures, junctions, and venous valves, and vein diameter increase the possibility of tip contact with the vein wall. This contact disrupts the endothelial cell layer of the tunica intima, exposes the basement membrane, and triggers the clotting process. If it is positioned to abut the vessel wall, physical as well as chemical damage are likely to result, increasing the risk of thrombosis. (Fletcher 2000) (Figure 12.9).*

Route of access

There continues to be debate as to which route of access carries the lowest risk of catheter-related thrombosis. Some studies demonstrate a lowest risk with the subclavian approach (Timsit *et al.* 1998); however, multiple studies have shown the opposite, that subclavian venous catheterisation results in a much higher incidence of venous stenosis and thrombosis than does catheterisation via the internal jugular approach (Cimochowski *et al.* 1990, Macdonald *et al.* 2000, Terotola 2000). Smaller bore dilators and catheters made from softer materials should reduce trauma to the vein on insertion and during subsequent use of the catheter.

Preferential use of the larger, proximal basilic vein rather than the cephalic vein for PICC insertion may also help to reduce the risk (Allen *et al.* 2000). Secure fixation of the device to the patient's skin will minimise movement of the catheter within the vein, once the PICC is in situ (Mazzola *et al.* 1999).

Anticoagulation

Intraluminal thrombosis may be prevented by adhering to appropriate flushing protocols as described elsewhere (see Chapter 14); however, this will have little impact on extraluminal thrombosis. Over the years in longer-term patients, it has become common

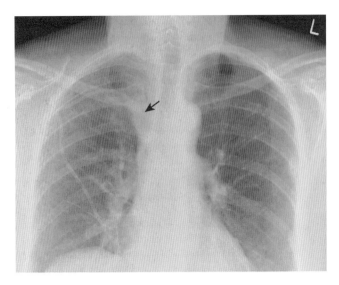

Figure 12.9 A Hickman catheter inserted via the right axillary subclavian route was initially in a satisfactory position in the SVC. Later it was malfunctioning and blood could not be aspirated. A chest X-ray shows the line has migrated outwards and the tip (arrow) is lying in an unsatisfactory position at the junction of the subclavian and innominate vein. This catheter needs removal and resiting elsewhere.

practice to use low-dose warfarin, e.g. 1 mg daily, which is usually a sub-therapeutic dose, to minimise the risk of thrombosis. Recent evidence, however, suggests that the use of low-dose warfarin has no apparent benefit for the prophylaxis of symptomatic catheter-related thrombosis in patients with cancer (Couban *et al.* 2005, Young *et al.* 2005). However, its use remains controversial and some clinicians may still continue to prescribe it. Therapeutic dose warfarin should be superior and some centres now use therapeutic dose low molecular weight heparin (Lee *et al.* 2005). Therapeutic dose anticoagulation increases the risk of bleeding, so is generally restricted to patients at very high risk or those who have had previous thromboembolic events.

Investigations

Contrast venography is the standard diagnostic tool for thrombosis (Lee and Levine 2000) but has an associated morbidity and may not always be available. The most effective non-invasive diagnostic method is compression or duplex ultrasound, which has been shown to be highly accurate in diagnosing deep vein thrombosis in leg veins (Lee and Levine 2000), and it would seem reasonable to expect a similar degree of accuracy in accessible veins in the upper body. Ultrasound cannot be used to visualise veins in the mediastinum unless a trans-oesophageal probe is used.

Management

Optimal management of CVC-related thrombosis is not clear (Lee and Levine 2000). Immediate removal of the catheter has been seen by some as the best option, but others argue that in cases where the patient has an ongoing need for central venous access, removal of the catheter will expose the patient to all the complications associated with reinsertion, including, of course, thrombosis. Kenney *et al.* (1996) report a 78% success rate in resolving the clinical symptoms of CVC-related thrombosis in paediatric patients by means of anticoagulation without catheter removal. Lee and Levine (2000) also advocate leaving the catheter in situ but argue that many questions remain to be answered including the optimal method of anticoagulation, and the relative merits of local or systemic thrombolysis versus anticoagulation.

Mechanical phlebitis

Definition and causes

Several authors writing about PICCs have described a phenomenon known as 'mechanical phlebitis'. Todd (1998) describes: 'pain, redness, warmth, a venous cord (a hard, palpable, thrombosed vein), induration and swelling' along the path of the vein usually within 14 days of PICC insertion.

The relationship between mechanical phlebitis and thrombosis is not generally discussed in the literature and does not appear to have been studied. Most authors treat the two complications separately. In a study of 1000 patients with PICCs, Ng *et al.* (1997) used two separate classifications: (1) Mechanical phlebitis showing 'tenderness, warmth or erythema (or some combination of these findings) at the site of insertion of the PICC or along the course of the vein, which occurred within 7 days of insertion and resolved without antibiotic therapy'. (2) Thrombosis showing 'generalized swelling of the extremity without signs of local infection or mechanical phlebitis which resulted in duplex scanning being carried out to confirm the diagnosis'. It is not known what duplex scanning might have revealed in those patients in the mechanical phlebitis group.

The risk factors for mechanical phlebitis appear to be remarkably similar to those for thrombosis, suggesting that mechanical phlebitis may in fact simply be an early stage of thrombosis. In a study of 128 patients with PICCs, Mazzola *et al.* (1999) found that the risk of mechanical phlebitis was increased in the following situations: (a) when larger gauge catheters were used, (b) if catheters were placed in the cephalic rather than the larger basilic vein, (c) the catheter tip was placed outside the SVC, (d) when there was manipulation or movement at the exit site.

Prevention

The risk of mechanical phlebitis should be reduced by attending to the above measures. Mazzola *et al.* (1999) also suggests the use of prophylactic heat therapy to dilate the vein, and improve blood flow, but the effectiveness of this strategy has yet to be studied. The author's own experience suggests an effective strategy in preventing mechanical phlebitis (as well as thrombosis) is to place the PICC in the upper arm (Figure 12.10). This is usually only possible with the use of ultrasound but has

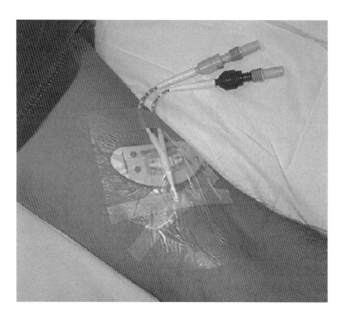

Figure 12.10 PICC with access site in upper arm vein rather than at the level of the elbow skin crease.

the effect of minimising movement of the catheter within the arm veins and therefore reducing the irritation which leads to mechanical phlebitis and thrombosis. The use of this technique has virtually eliminated phlebitis in PICC patients at the author's institution.

Management

Various authors suggest the use of heat therapy when mechanical phlebitis occurs (Aston 2000). Todd (1998) also advises elevation of the arm, gentle exercise, increased fluid intake and analgesia until the phlebitis resolves.

Incorrect catheter tip position

A CVC should be considered to be in an incorrect position when any of the following apply:

- The tip of the device is in the venous system but not correctly positioned in the right atrium, the SVC or the IVC.
- The distal section and tip of the catheter is not lying parallel to the vein wall.
- The line is kinked within the body or pinched between internal structures.
- The catheter lies outside the venous system.

Catheters within the venous system

Incorrect or suboptimal catheter position is common during blind placement of catheters particularly from the subclavian or left-sided routes due to the necessity to traverse corners. Tortuous veins, vein stenosis, abnormal anatomy and poor insertion technique are other relevant factors. Typical examples and some solutions are shown in Chapter 11, and most are easily repositioned with screening at the time or soon after insertion. Providing such malposition is recognised, usually no problems ensue. If such problems are identified later then a decision will be required as to the future of the catheter.

Incorrect position may occur in a previously well-positioned device. The catheter may become dislodged if it is not correctly secured in place, or is accidentally pulled out, displacing the internal tip of the device (Figure 12.9). In tunnelled catheters and implantable ports, positioning the exit site within mobile tissue (e.g. large breasts) can also lead to movement of the whole catheter and displacement of the tip. In ports, this may lead to kinking or even breakage of the tunnelled portion of the device. In addition, it is not unknown for a catheter to 'migrate' within the venous system for no apparent reason. Hadaway (1998) reports that 'Changes in intrathoracic pressure, coughing, sneezing, a Valsalva manoeuvre such as during heavy lifting, vigorous extremity use, forceful flushing, or congestive heart failure could lead to migration of the tip'.

The consequences of leaving a malpositioned catheter in place may be serious. If the tip of the catheter moves to a vessel other than the SVC/IVC or the right atrium, the risk of thrombosis (and by implication subsequent infection) is increased significantly. This is because other veins are more convoluted, smaller and have less blood flow, allowing chemical and mechanical damage to the vein wall to occur much more easily. Typically, for catheters inserted by the subclavian or left internal jugular, a poorly placed catheter tip may abut the sidewall of the SVC at an acute angle (see Chapter 2). In addition, infusion of fluids and/or drugs via a malpositioned catheter may lead to great vein perforation (see section above) and extravasation. Multiple lumen catheters are at particular risk for this problem. Where drugs such as vesicant chemotherapy are involved, the consequences for the patient can be extremely serious (see below).

Recognition

Incorrect position should be suspected clinically in the event of

- Patency problems which persist despite the use of a thrombolytic.
- Discomfort during flushing with/without signs of extravasation of drugs/fluids.
- Signs of the catheter 'ballooning' beneath skin during flushing (tunnelled lines).
- An increase in the length of the external portion of the catheter. In a tunnelled CVC, the Dacron 'cuff' may protrude out of the exit site and become visible.
- The development of a thrombosis.
- Failure to measure CVP or monitor the CVP trace.

Incorrect positioning may be obvious on plain X-rays, but the limitations of plain films should be appreciated (see Chapter 2). If there is doubt about the position of the catheter then X-ray contrast injected through the catheter with fluoroscopy will identify its position within venous, arterial or extravascular positions.

Management

In most circumstances, a malpositioned, kinked or pinched catheter should be repositioned, replaced or removed as soon as practicable. For short-term catheters used for fluid infusion or monitoring CVP or in emergency situations, it may be reasonable to withdraw the catheter until blood can be aspirated freely, check the catheter position radiologically and clinically, and use the catheter cautiously. In the longer-term catheter, the risk benefits of radiological repositioning a misplaced catheter (see Chapter 10) versus resiting from a new entry site need to be balanced in the individual patient. Leaving misplaced catheters in place for any length of time represents a high risk of thrombosis and/or catheter fracture/embolism (Aitkin and Minton 1984).

Catheters outside the venous system

This is a potentially dangerous situation and catheters have been reported lying in just about every anatomical location possible including the arterial tree, respiratory system, pleural space, mediastinum (Figure 12.8), pericardium, peritoneal space, liver and other viscera. Careful consideration should be given as to the safest means of removal as discussed in the sections above.

Embolised, fractured or irretrievable guidewires and catheters

Catheter fracture may occur due to accidental cutting of the line, or repeated clamping outside a designated clamping area. In tunnelled CVCs, there is the added possibility of internal fracture due to pinching or kinking of a badly positioned catheter. A phenomenon known as 'pinch-off' can occur with subclavian catheters (Aitkin and Minton 1984), where the catheter is pinched between the clavicle and first rib. This may be predicted if the catheter is blocked/unblocked by shoulder movements. In such cases, the catheter should be removed as the risk of catheter fracture is high (see Chapters 7 and 15). In implantable ports, the port and catheter may in rare cases become detached from one another (Moore *et al.* 1986).

Internal fracture carries a risk of catheter embolism. Fragments of catheter will typically migrate centrally to the SVC, right atrium, right ventricle or pulmonary arteries and should be removed wherever possible to reduce the risk of thrombus formation and infection. Catheters already in place may be perforated by needle placement for additional catheter placement.

External fracture is usually revealed by leakage of blood or fluids during flushing. The catheter should be clamped immediately to prevent air embolism and in many cases will need to be removed as soon as possible to prevent infection. If the right equipment and skills are available, the catheter can often be repaired using a dedicated repair kit.

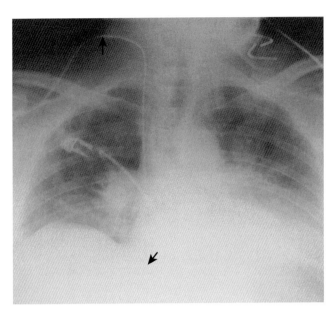

Figure 12.11 A lost guidewire initially went unnoticed after right internal jugular insertion procedure by an inexperienced trainee, although one lumen of the multiple lumen catheter was blocked. When the catheter was removed, fortunately the lost guidewire came out with it, much to the surprise of staff. Retrospective review of the chest X-ray showed the radiopaque wire with proximal end in situ in one lumen of the catheter above the right collarbone. The wire passes downwards off the chest X-ray into the inferior vena cava (arrow).

The infection risk posed by repairing and leaving a potentially contaminated catheter in situ should be weighed against the possible complications of inserting a new CVC.

Internal fracture should be suspected if there is pain, redness or swelling on flushing or administration of fluids. The patency of the catheter may also be impaired. In cases where the catheter has fractured completely and catheter embolism has occurred, the patient may exhibit signs of pulmonary embolism. A catheter that has fractured internally should be removed or replaced as soon as possible and the internal fragment retrieved surgically or radiologically (see Chapter 12 for further information).

Rare complications involving Seldinger wires are repeatedly cited in the literature. Guidewire embolisation can occur when inexperienced operators fail to keep hold to the guidewire during catheter insertion (see Figure 12.10). Seldinger wires can become tethered within a vessel, usually within one of the neck veins. This occurs mainly in patients with abnormal vessels. There are repeated incidents of wires that have become kinked or knotted (Burns *et al.* 1989, Carpentier *et al.* 1991). Similar problems are seen with catheters which may kink, knot or get tangled with other devices. Long-term catheters may become permanently tethered by clot and fibrin sleeves to the central veins or right atrial wall. This may be a particular problem with catheters with multiple side holes (e.g. apheresis catheters) where organised clot gets trapped within the multiples holes.

Such cases may be resolved by attempts to dilate the venous system, e.g. by asking a conscious patient to perform the Valsalva manoeuvre, or by increasing the patient's

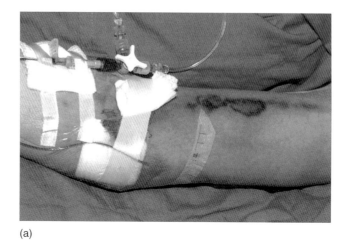

(a)

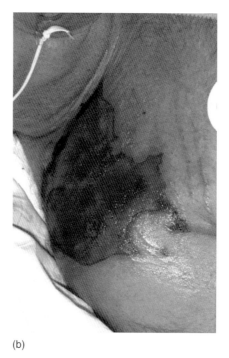

(b)

Figure 12.12 (a) Extravasation injury is common with cancer chemotherapy as shown here in the upper arm with a PICC inserted to bypass the area. (b) Severe extravasation injury with extensive tissue necrosis following leakage of amiodarone and noradrenaline into the deeper tissues around a subclavian catheter. Debridement and skin grafting was required.

circulating volume by peripheral administration of additional intravenous fluids. The patient's vital signs should be monitored closely and the Trendelenburg position maintained throughout. If these techniques are unsuccessful then interventional radiology or surgical removal will be required (see also Chapters 7, 10 and 15). There is a place for leaving such catheters fragments in situ if removal is impractical or dangerous, this is most commonly seen in the case of permanent pacemaker leads which become anchored to the myocardium (see Chapter 11).

Extravasation injury

Extravasation is very common and is a major reason for removal of 'tissued' peripheral cannulae. If the infused drug or solution is relatively isotonic, no serious sequelae usually follow. The situation with leakage of hypertonic, sclerosant solutions is very different and is one reason why many drugs and solutions are recommended only for central vein administration. Common examples are cancer chemotherapy drugs, vasopressor agents, calcium chloride, sodium bicarbonate and amiodarone. Leakage of such agents into the tissues commonly causes severe phlebitis and superficial damage in the limbs but can cause more severe necrosis if leakage occurs in the deeper tissues around a central catheter (see Figures 12.11a and 12.11b). Close attention to detail to ensure catheters of an adequate length and are in the correct position (see above) is essential to avoid such problems. Short catheters inserted into the femoral vessels may be a particular risk as they are easily dislodged if the hip is flexed (Figure 12.12). If problems occur then any residual fluid should be aspirated from the catheter and tissues. The catheter should be left temporarily in position to consider if there is potential benefit to injection of agents to neutralise the extravasated solution. Pharmacy departments stock various agents for this purpose. It should be appreciated that the proximal port(s) of a multilumen catheter may be extravascular whilst the distal port remains in the vein if the catheter migrates outwards.

Conclusion

CVCs play a vital role in management of patients in a wide variety of healthcare settings. Many modern treatments would be impossible without them and without doubt they have helped save many lives and improved the quality of many others. However, it is important to remember that CVCs are associated with significant morbidity and occasional mortality. It is vital that those who insert and manage CVCs are educated in the wide range of complications associated with their use.

References

Aggarwal P, Hari P, Bagga A *et al.* (2000). Phrenic nerve palsy: a rare complication of indwelling subclavian vein catheter. *Pediatric Nephrology* 14:203–204.

Aitkin DR, Minton JP (1984). The 'Pinch-off Sign': a warning of impending problems with permanent subclavian catheters. *American Journal of Surgery* 148:633–636.

Allen AW, Megargell JL, Brown DB *et al.* (2000). Venous thrombosis associated with the placement of peripherally inserted central catheters. *Journal of Vascular and Interventional Radiology* 11:1309–1314.

Alomari A, Falk A (2006). Median nerve bisection: a morbid complication of a peripherally inserted central catheter. *Journal of Vascular Access* 7:129–131.

Aston V (2000). Community management of peripherally inserted central catheters. *British Journal of Community Nursing* 5:318–325.

Balestreri L, De Cicco M, Matovic M *et al.* (1995). Central venous catheter-related thrombosis in clinically asymptomatic oncologic patients: a phlebographic study. *European Journal of Radiology* 20:108–111.

Barnacle A, Kleidon T (2005). Lymphatic leak complicating central venous catheter insertion. *Cardiovascular and Interventional Radiology* 28:839–840.

Belcaster A (1997). Venous air embolism. *Nursing* 27:33.

Bivins MH, Callahan MJ (2000). Position-dependent ventricular tachycardia related to a peripherally inserted central catheter. *Mayo Clinic Proceedings* 75:414–416.

Blot F, Nitenberg G, Brun-Buisson C (2000). New tools in diagnosing catheter-related infections. *Supportive Care in Cancer* 8:287–292.

Brothers TE, Von Moll LK, Niederhuber JA *et al.* (1988). Experience with subcutaneous infusion ports in three hundred patients. *Surgery Gynecology and Obstetrics* 166:295–301.

Burns AM, Shelly MP, Abbott TR (1989). Kinking of a Seldinger Wire. *Anaesthesia* 44:267.

Carpentier JP, Braz SJ, Choukroun G *et al.* (1991). Formation of a knot in a J spiral metallic guide: a complication of the Seldinger method. *Cahiers D Anesthesiologie* 39:8.

Cartwright DW (2002). Placement of neonatal central venous catheter tips: is the right atrium so dangerous? *Archives of Disease in Childhood Fetal and Neonatal Edition* 87:F155–F156.

Caruso L, Gravenstein N, Layon AJ *et al.* (2003). Central venous catheter tip and perforation. *Anesthesia and Analgesia* 96:301–302.

Cimochowski G, Worley E, Rutherford WE *et al.* (1990). Superiority of the internal jugular over subclavian access for temporary dialysis. *Nephron* 54:154–161.

Cornock M (1996). Making sense of CVCs. *Nursing Times* 92:30–31.

Couban S, Goodyear M, Burnell M *et al.* (2005). Randomised placebo controlled study of low-dose warfarin for the prevention of central venous catheter associated thrombosis in patients with cancer. *Journal of Clinical Oncology* 20:4063–4069.

Dobbins BM, Catton JA, Kite P *et al.* (2003). Each lumen is a potential source of central venous catheter-related bloodstream infection. *Critical Care Medicine* 31:1688–1690.

Dougherty L, Lister SE (2004). Vascular access devices. In *Manual of Clinical Nursing Procedures*, 6th edn, Dougherty L, Lister S (eds), Blackwell Science, Oxford, UK.

Drewett S (2000a). Complications of central venous catheters: nursing care. *British Journal of Nursing* 9:466–478.

Drewett S (2000b). Central venous catheter removal: procedures and rationale. *British Journal of Nursing* 9:2304–2315.

Fitchet A, Fitzpatrick AP (1998). Central venous air embolism causing pulmonary oedema mimicking left ventricular failure. *BMJ* 316:604–606.

Flaccadori E, Gonzi G, Zambrelli G *et al.* (1996). Cardiac arrhythmias during central venous catheter procedures in acute renal failure: a prospective study. *Journal of the American Society of Nephrology* 7:1079–1084.

Fletcher SJ, Bodenham AR (2000). Editorial II: Safe placement of central venous catheters: where should the tip of the catheter lie? *British Journal of Anaesthesia* 85:188–191.

Grove J, Pevec W (2000). Venous thrombosis related to peripherally inserted central catheters. *Journal of Vascular and Interventional Radiology* 11:837–840.

Hadaway L (1998). Major thrombotic and non-thrombotic complications: loss of patency. *Journal of Intravenous Nursing* 21:S143–S160.

Hall K, Farr B (2004). Diagnosis and management of long-term central venous catheter infections. *Journal of Vascular Interventional Radiology* 15:327–334.

Haller L, Rush K (1992). CVC infection: a review. *Journal of Clinical Nursing* 1:61–66.

Horowitz MD, Alkire MJ, Lickstein DA *et al.* (1991). Aortic injury as a complication of central venous catheterization. *American Heart Journal* 122:595–597.

Kayley J (1997). Skin-tunnelled cuffed catheters. *Community Nurse* 3:21–22.

Kenney BD, David M, Bensoussan AL *et al.* (1996). Anticoagulation without catheter removal in children with catheter- related central vein thrombosis. *Journal of Pediatric Surgery* 31:816–818.

Kite P, Dobbins BM, Wilcox MH *et al.* (1997). Evaluation of a novel endoluminal brush method for in situ diagnosis of catheter related sepsis. *Journal of Clinical Pathology* 50:278–282.

Krzywda EA (2002). Central venous catheter infections: clinical aspects of microbial etiology and pathogenesis. *Journal of Infusion Nursing* 25:29–35.

Latto IP, Ng WS, Jones PL *et al.* (2000). *Percutaneous Central Venous and Arterial Catheterisation*, 3rd edn, WB Saunders, London, UK.

Lee A, Levine M (2000). Management of venous thromboembolism in cancer patients. *Oncology* 14:409–417.

Lee AYY, Rickles FR, Julian JA *et al.* (2005). Randomised comparison of low molecular weight heparin and coumarin derivatives on survival of patients with cancer and thromboembolism. *Journal of Clinical Oncology* 23:2123–2130.

Lee T-Y, Sun CS, Chu YC *et al.* (1996). Incidence and risk factors of guidewire-induced arrhythmia during internal jugular venous catheterization: comparison of marked and plain J-wires. *Journal of Clinical Anesthesia* 8:348–351.

Lemmer JH, Zwischenberger JB, Bove EL *et al.* (1987). Lymph leak from a femoral cut down site in a neonate repair with fibrin glue. *Journal Paediatric Surgery* 22:827–828.

Macdonald S, Watt AJ, McNally D *et al.* (2000). Comparison of technical success and outcome of tunnelled catheters inserted via the jugular and subclavian approaches. *Journal of Vascular and Interventional Radiology* 11:225–231.

Mallick A, Bodenham AR (2003). Disorders of the lymph circulation: their relevance to anaesthesia and intensive care. *British Journal of Anaesthesia* 91:265–272.

Marinella MA, Kathula SK, Markert RJ *et al.* (2000). Spectrum of upper-extremity deep venous thrombosis in a community teaching hospital. *Heart and Lung: The Journal of Acute and Critical Care* 29:113–117.

Mazzola JR, Schott-Baer D, Addy L *et al.* (1999). Clinical factors associated with the development of phlebitis after insertion of a peripherally inserted central catheter. *Journal of Intravenous Nursing* 22:36–42.

McCarthy P (1995). Air embolism in single-lung transplant patients after central venous catheter removal. *Chest* 107:1178–1179.

Mercer-Jones MA, Wenstone R, Hershman MJ *et al.* (1995). Fatal subclavian artery haemorrhage. A complication of subclavian vein catheterisation. *Anaesthesia* 50:639–640.

Merry AF, Webster CS, van Cotthem IC *et al.* (1999). A prospective randomized clinical assessment of a new pigtail central venous catheter in comparison with standard alternatives. *Anaesthesia and Intensive Care* 27:639–645.

Moore C *et al.* (1986). Nursing care and management of venous access ports. *Oncology Nursing Forum* 13:35–39.

Ng PK, Ault MJ, Ellrodt AG *et al.* (1997). Peripherally inserted central catheters in general medicine. *Mayo Clinic Proceedings* 72:225–233.

NICE (National Institute for Clinical Excellence) (2002). *Guidance on the Use of Ultrasound Locating Devices for Placing Central Venous Catheters*. NICE Technology Appraisal No 49. London, UK. Available at www.nice.org.uk

Nowicka M, Wiatr E, Kupis W *et al.* (2004). Respiratory distress and peritonitis after femoral vein cannulation in a 1.5 year-old child. Case report. *Anestezjologia Intensywna Terapia* 36:282–285.

Orme RM, McSwiney MM, Chamberlain-Webber RFO *et al.* (2007). Fatal cardiac tamponade as a result of a peripherally inserted central venous catheter: a case report and review of the literature. *British Journal of Anaesthesia* 99:384–388.

Parikh S, Narayanan V (2004). Misplaced peripherally inserted central catheter: an unusual cause of stroke. *Pediatric Neurology* 30:210–212.

Perdue MB (2001). Intravenous complications. In *Infusion Therapy in Clinical Practice*, 2nd edn, Carlson K, Perdue MB, Hankins J (eds), WB Saunders, Pennsylvania, PA.

Pratt RJ, Pellowe CM, Wilson JA *et al.* (2007). EPIC2: National evidence-based guidelines for preventing healthcare-associated infections in NHS. *Journal of Hospital Infection* 65:S1–S59.

Quiney NF (1994). Sudden death after central venous cannulation. *Canadian Journal of Anaesthesia* 41:513–515.

Racadio JM, Doellman DA, Johnson ND *et al.* (2001). Pediatric peripherally inserted central catheters: complication rates related to catheter tip location. *Pediatrics* 107:E28.

Reed GL, Houng AK (1999). The contribution of activated factor XIII to fibrinolytic resistance in experimental pulmonary embolism. *Circulation* 99:299–304.

Reuber M, Dunkley LA, Gusmano F *et al.* (2002). Stroke after internal jugular venous cannulation. *Acta Neurologica Scandinavica* 105:235–239.

Ricci M, Puente AO, Gusmano F *et al.* (1999). Central venous access: accidental arterial puncture in a patient with right-sided aortic arch. *Critical Care Medicine* 27:1025–1026.

Robinson JF, Robinson WA, Cohn A *et al.* (1995). Perforation of the great vessels during central venous line placement. *Archives of Internal Medicine* 155:1225–1228.

Robinson JL (2002). Sensitivity of a blood culture drawn through a single lumen of a multilumen, long-term, indwelling, central venous catheter in pediatric oncology patients. *Journal of Pediatric Hematology/Oncology* 24:72–74.

Ross VM (2003). Uncertainty about the clinical detection of sepsis. *Journal of Infusion Nursing* 26:23–28.

Russell WC, Greiff J (2003). Fatal cardiac perforation by central venous catheter dilators: does the length matter? *Anaesthesia* 58:1241–1242.

Safdar N, Maki D (2002). Inflammation at the insertion site is not predictive of catheter-related bloodstream infection with short-term, noncuffed central venous catheters. *Critical Care Medicine* 30:2632–2635.

Stuart RK, Baxter JK, Shikora SA *et al.* (1992). Reducing arrhythmias associated with central venous catheter insertion or exchange. *Nutrition* 8:19–21.

Terotola SO (2000). Haemodilaysis catheter placement and management. *Radiology* 215:651–658.

Tighe M, Kite P, Fawley WN *et al.* (1996). An endoluminal brush to detect the infected central venous catheter in situ: a pilot study. *BMJ* 14:313–317.

Timsit JF, Misset B, Carlet J *et al.* (1998). Central vein catheter-related thrombosis in intensive care patients: incidence, risk factors and relationship with catheter-related sepsis. *Chest* 114:207–213.

Todd J (1998). Peripherally inserted central catheters. *Professional Nurse* 13:297–302.

Vesely T (2003). Central venous catheter tip position: a continuing controversy. *Journal of Vascular and Interventional Radiology* 14:527–534.

Vesely TM (2001). Air embolism during insertion of central venous catheters. *Journal of Vascular and Interventional Radiology* 12:1291–1295.

Wariyar UK, Hallworth D (June 2001). *Review of Four Neonatal Deaths due to Cardiac Tamponade Associated with the Presence of a Central Venous Catheter: Recommendations and Department of Health Response.* Available at www.medical-devices.gov.uk.

Weinstein SM (2001). *Plumer's Principles and Practice of Infusion Therapy*, 7th edn. Lippincott Williams and Wilkins, Philadelphia, PA.

Wysoki MG (2001). Evaluation of various manoeuvres for prevention of air embolism during central venous catheter placement. *Journal of Vascular and Interventional Radiology* 12:764–766.

Young AM, Begum G, Billingham LJ *et al.* (2005) WARP – a multicentre prospective randomised controlled trial (RCT) of thrombosis prophylaxis with warfarin in cancer patients with central venous catheters (CVCs).

Zsolt AV, Gyor-Molnar I, Kollar L *et al.* (2002). A surgically treated arteriovenous fistula between the vertebral artery and internal jugular vein after insertion of a central venous catheter for mitral valve replacement. *Journal of Thoracic and Cardiovascular Surgery* 123:575–577.

Chapter 13

The pathogenesis and prevention of intravascular catheter-related infections

T.S.J. Elliott

Introduction

The majority of hospital-acquired bacteraemias and septicaemias are related to the use of intravascular catheters, with the incidence of catheter-related bloodstream infections ranging from 2 to 14 episodes per thousand catheter days (Arnow *et al.* 1993, Eggimann and Pittet 2002). Infection rates vary widely and depend on various factors including the patient's underlying condition, the duration of catheter insertion, the site of catheterisation as well as the type of catheter used and the degree of aseptic precautions taken (Elliott 2001). The rate of catheter-related bloodstream infections for peripherally inserted catheters is lower than that for central venous catheters (CVCs) (Elliott 1988). In this chapter, prevention of catheter-related infection focuses on central venous devices.

Types of intravascular catheter-related infections

Infections associated with intravascular catheters can be divided into two main groups: localised or systemic. Localised infections involve the exit site of the catheter and should ideally be diagnosed early with regular observations of the insertion site being an essential component of catheter care. Localised infections may present with erythema, oedema and a purulent exudate. This should be distinguished from clear exudates, which commonly occur following catheter insertion. Localised infections may also involve thrombophlebitis within the cannulated blood vessel or subcutaneous sepsis which are associated with tunnelled devices. Cellulitis can occasionally spread from the catheter exit site, particularly when the causative microorganisms are *Streptococcus pyogenes* or *Staphylococcus aureus*. In comparison, a patient who has a systemic infection associated with intravascular catheters may have a low-grade pyrexia usually <38.5°C with no other obvious source of infection (Elliott 1988). The patient may also have a transient pyrexia or rigour following flushing of the device. In addition, patients commonly have positive blood cultures from which a microorganism recognised as causing catheter sepsis is isolated. Ideally, blood cultures should be obtained through the catheter as well as a separate peripheral venepuncture and if both are culture positive with the same microorganism this can assist in confirming the diagnosis. The laboratory methods to establish the diagnosis of catheter-related sepsis have been recently extensively reviewed (Worthington and Elliott 2005). The methods reviewed included catheter brushing, leucocyte cytospin on blood obtained via the CVC and serology. Differential timing to positive testing between peripheral versus central catheter cultures has also been suggested as a technique to diagnose catheter-related sepsis. However, paired blood cultures obtained via the catheter and also from a separate peripheral venepuncture without differential timing are still the recommended approach for routine microbiology laboratories.

A clinical response to empirical antimicrobial therapy or following catheter removal will also support the diagnosis. Catheter-related infections may, however, be unresponsive to broad-spectrum antibiotics and require catheter removal. The management of catheter-related infections has also been recently reviewed and guidelines presented for when catheters should be removed (Elliott 2004). Culture of the explanted catheter distal tip and isolation of the same microorganisms as from blood cultures can confirm the diagnosis. It is important to remove catheters when certain infections such as those caused by *S. aureus* or *Candida* spp. are diagnosed. This reduces the likelihood of relapses and re-infections.

Sources of microorganisms resulting in catheter-related infections

There are five routes by which microorganisms may gain access to the indwelling catheter surface resulting eventually in catheter tip colonisation and subsequent bacteraemia and septicaemia (Elliott 2000).These are summarised in Box 13.1, and discussed below.

1. *Extraluminal*: Microorganisms may gain access to catheters via extraluminal route along the outside surface of the device. The microorganisms are usually derived from the patients own skin microflora. This source of infection is primarily related to the inability of currently available skin antiseptics to sterilise the skin at the

---

Box 13.1 Sources of microorganisms which cause catheter-related infection:

1. Extraluminal – via outside of catheter surface
2. Intraluminal – via internal luminal spread
3. Haematogenous – via blood stream
4. Contamination of fluids or drugs – via giving set
5. Impaction – at the time of insertion

site of catheter insertion. Sub-optimal skin antiseptic preparations or inadequate methods of application may also exacerbate this problem. For example, the use of preparations containing alcohol should always be allowed adequate time to dry before catheter insertion is attempted. This can take up to 2 minutes and is commonly not complied with. Similarly, techniques such as poor surgical asepsis, the use of inappropriate dressings which encourage microbial multiplication, use of wet shaving with a blade may result in the skin catheter insertion site becoming a source of microorganisms. Infection may then develop at this site. Microorganisms derived either from the skin insertion site or from any local infection may then transverse along the outer surface of the catheter tract until they reach the intravascular distal tip. If a device is tunnelled, an associated tunnel infection may also occur. Once colonisation of a catheter develops, this can then act as a source of bacteraemia and septicaemia. Catheter insertion site sepsis does not have to occur before septicaemia develops.

2. *Intraluminal*: Microorganisms have been shown to colonise the internal components of catheter hubs as well as the internal surface of luer connectors (Tebbs *et al.* 1996). The opening of the closed catheter system, for example when a luer is connected to a giving set so that fluids can be given to a patient, may result in internal microbial contamination followed by intraluminal migration of microorganisms. Luers can readily become contaminated with microorganisms. For example, it has been shown that 23% of luers are contaminated in the intensive care unit setting within 3 days of catheter insertion (Salzman 1993, Tebbs *et al.* 1996).

   Sitges-Serra (1997) further demonstrated that colonised hubs are a likely source of catheter-related septicaemia and that microorganisms can migrate along the internal catheter surface resulting in colonisation and sepsis. Indeed, this route is thought to be responsible for the highest proportion of catheter-related bloodstream infections in patients with long-term CVC (Linares *et al.* 1985).

3. *Haematogenous*: The spread of microorganisms via the bloodstream commonly referred to as haematogenous seeding can result in microorganisms gaining access to a catheter surface (Eggimann and Pittet 2002). This source of microorganism is less common as compared to the endoluminal and extraluminal routes (Pearson 1996).

4. *Contamination of fluids or drugs*: Contaminated infusions may also result in catheter-related sepsis (Henderson 1988, Maki 1992). Infusates may be contaminated during manufacturing or when manipulating intravenous giving sets to attach to catheters or even when preparing fluids for injection. This overall relatively rare source of microorganisms may also result in catheter colonisation and associated sepsis.

5. *Impaction at the time of insertion*: Another potentially overlooked source of contamination is also from the patients own skin microflora as with extraluminal contamination. However, this occurs when the catheter is inserted through the patient's skin and microorganisms present at this site are impacted onto the catheter distal surface tip during the procedure (Elliott 1997). In a unique study, we investigated patients undergoing open heart surgery following the insertion of a CVC. When the distal tips of the catheters were sampled in situ within 1 hour of implantation, microorganisms were detected on the catheters surface in 17% of patients. This

potential source of sepsis offers an explanation for the presence of microorganisms predominantly on the catheter distal tips and again illustrates the importance of skin antisepsis.

Development of catheter-related sepsis

When microorganisms gain access to the catheter surface, they can attach directly onto the polymer and produce a biofilm which consists of a complex polysaccharide called glycocalyx. This biofilm assists in protecting the microorganisms from immunological defences including neutrophil action, and can also limit antibiotic penetration making these infections difficult to treat. Following insertion of an intravascular catheter into a patient, a biofilm, consisting of proteins and platelets, also rapidly forms on the polymer surface within a few hours. This can also result in entrapment of microorganisms and offers further binding sites such as fibronectin which is used for attachment of some staphylococci.

Causative microorganisms of catheter-related infections

The majority of microorganisms implicated in catheter-related infections are derived from the patients own skin microflora and are shown in Table 13.1 (Elliott 1988).

The Gram-positive cocci including *S. aureus* and the coagulase-negative staphylococci such as *Staphylococcus epidermidis* are the predominant causes of catheter-related infections. Gram-negative bacilli and in particular, coliforms (Enterobacteriaceae) are mainly related to patients located in higher risk areas such as intensive care units. In particular, the coliforms as a cause of catheter-related sepsis are associated with patients who are ventilated with a tracheostomy site which are colonised with these microorganisms (Elliott TSJ, unpublished data). Colonisation of the upper respiratory airways has also been shown to be a risk factor in these patients (Pittet *et al.* 1995). Interestingly, *Candida* species have become an important pathogen and have been reported in a range of patients including those located on intensive care units, patients who are receiving total parenteral nutrition, or immunosuppressive drugs such as steroids.

Table 13.1 Range of microorgansims (as a percentage) causing catheter-related infection.

Microorganism	Approximate percentage
Coagulase-negative staphylococci	60–70
Staphylococcus aureus	15
Methicillin-resistant *Staphylococcus aureus*	< 5
Candida species	< 5.0
Enterococci	2–4
Enterobacteriaceae (coliforms)	5–10

Prevention of intravascular catheter-related infections

The logical approach to the prevention of these catheter-related infections is to consider three areas: the device, the patient and the health care worker. These are considered below.

The device

Several approaches have been taken in order to prevent intravascular catheter-related infections. These include redesigning catheter components, formation of new coatings and polymers with fewer plasticisers and with a smoother surface. Improvements in the skin penetrative properties of introducer needles have also been achieved by redesigning the needle bevel to allow penetration through the skin with a minimum amount of trauma. This reduces the likelihood of sepsis by resulting in less tissue damage and exudate formation and therefore facilitates healing. Anti-adhesive coatings have also been developed. These include hydromers which have been used to coat catheters. Such hydrophilic materials have been shown to reduce colonisation in in vitro studies (Tebbs and Elliott 1994).

More recently, antimicrobial catheters have been developed in an attempt to act as prophylactic agents to stop catheters becoming colonised resulting in infection. A range of antimicrobial agents have been tested (Elliott 1997, 1999). The most comprehensively studied antimicrobial catheters which are available for clinical use are those which have been coated with a combination of minocycline and rifampicin or chlorhexidine and silver sulphadiazine. These are discussed in detail below.

(i) *Minocycline–rifampicin-coated catheters*: The efficacy of these catheters for the prevention of catheter colonisation and sepsis has been studied in several trials (Raad *et al*. 1997, Marik *et al*. 1999, Chatzinikolaou *et al*. 2003, Leon *et al*. 2004, Hanna *et al*. 2004). In a double blind randomised clinical trial 281 hospitalised patients received either the antimicrobial-coated or uncoated catheter (Raad *et al*. 1997). Colonisation occurred in 36 (26%) of uncoated catheters compared to 11 (8%) of coated catheters. A significant reduction ($p < 0.001$) in microbial colonisation was achieved. Of more importance, catheter-related bloodstream infections were also significantly reduced ($p < 0.001$) with seven patients who had uncoated catheters and none with coated catheters developing bacteraemia. Indeed, in recent meta-analysis by our group, the use of such antimicrobial CCV was found to be associated with a significant reduction in colonisation and catheter-related bloodstream infection (Casey *et al*. 2008). In another multi-centre clinical trial, the minocycline–rifampicin catheter was compared to a CVC-coated catheter with the antiseptic combination of chlorhexidine and silver sulphadiazine (Darouiche *et al*. 1999). A total of 738 catheters were studied and of these 356 were impregnated with minocycline and rifampicin and 382 with chlorhexidine and silver sulphadiazine. The catheters which contained minocycline and rifampicin were shown to be 3-fold less likely to be colonised and 12-fold less likely to be associated with catheter-related bloodstream infections than those coated with the chlorhexidine and silver sulphadiazine. Again, our meta-analysis of two studies demonstrated a significant reduction in the rate of both colonisation and catheter-related bloodstream infection associated with the use of the minocycline-rifampicin CVC (Darouiche *et al.* 1999, Marik *et al.* 1999, Casey *et al.* 2008).

The minocycline–rifampicin catheter retains its antimicrobial activity for at least 2 weeks in situ and would therefore appear to offer protection from microbial colonisation and infection during this period. A recent analysis suggests that CVCs coated with minocycline–rifampicin are cost-effective, particularly when patients are catheterised for at least 1 week (Marciante *et al.* 2003).

(ii) *Chlorhexidine and silver sulphadiazine coated catheters*: Chlorhexidine and silver sulphadiazine catheters are now available with coating of both the internal and external surface. The earlier devices were coated only on the external surfaces, which needs to be taken into account when assessing the early clinical trials. The antiseptics are released in vivo in approximately 15 days (Elliott 1999). The combination of chlorhexidine and the silver sulphadiazine has been shown to be active against a range of microorganisms (Maki *et al.* 1997, Marciante *et al.* 2003). The efficacy of these antimicrobial CVC has been studied in numerous clinical trials (Van Heerden *et al.* 1996, Bach *et al.* 1996, Pemberton *et al.* 1996, Ciresi *et al.* 1996, Tennenberg *et al.* 1997, Maki *et al.* 1997, Logghe *et al.* 1997, Heard *et al.* 1998, Marik *et al.* 1999, Hannan *et al.* 1999, Collin 1999, Sheng *et al.* 2000, Jaegar *et al.* 2005, Dunser *et al.* 2005, Osma *et al.* 2006). Indeed, Maki *et al.* (1997) carried out a comparative study with the chlorhexidine silver sulphadiazine catheters (72 patients with 208 catheters) compared to non-antimicrobial controlled devices (86 patients within 195 catheters). The number of colonised antimicrobial catheters was significantly reduced as compared to the control catheters (13.5% versus 24.1%, $p = 0.005$). In addition, the CVC-related bacteraemia rate was significantly reduced (1.0 versus 4.6%, $p = 0.03$). In our recent meta-analysis it was concluded that the chlorhexidine silver sulphadiazine was effective in reducing the incidence of both catheter colonisation and catheter-related sepsis in this group of patients (Casey *et al.* 2008). Chlorhexidine silver sulphadiazine impregnated catheters therefore offers a mechanism to reduce catheter-related infections particularly in settings where the relative incidence of associated sepsis is high (Maki *et al.* 1997).

Concern has been raised about the emergence of potential resistance to the antiseptic or antibiotic components of antimicrobials used in catheter polymers. This does not, however, appear to be a clinical problem. In the clinical trials to date, there have been no reported microbial resistance associated directly with the use of these catheters.

Anaphylactic reactions have, however, been associated with the use of chlorhexidine silver sulphadiazine impregnated catheters with 12 cases being reported in Japan (Oda *et al.* 1997), and more recently in a report from the UK (Stephens *et al.* 2001). This is a relatively rare side effect which health care workers need to be aware of. In summary, the use of CVCs impregnated with chlorhexidine silver sulphadiazine or rifampicin–minocycline should be considered when intravenous catheterisation is expected to be between 1 and 3 weeks and where the rate of infection is high despite implementation of preventative measures (Pratt *et al.* 2007).

Catheter hubs containing antiseptics

As discussed above, hubs can become contaminated with microorganisms, which then may act as a source of sepsis. Segura *et al.* (1996) have investigated the use of a catheter hub filled with iodine to overcome this source of sepsis. This antiseptic hub was shown to reduce the rate of catheter bloodstream infections as compared to standard non-antiseptic hubs. Other studies have, however, failed to show that this new hub prevents catheter-related sepsis (Luna *et al.* 2000). Further clinical trials are therefore required to enable this approach to be fully evaluated.

Needleless connectors

Needleless intravenous access devices have been developed in order to reduce the exposure of health care workers to needles, thereby reducing the likelihood of an inoculation injury (Trim and Elliott 2003). Several non-prospective, non-randomised clinical studies with these devices have, however, demonstrated an increased risk of catheter infections (Kellerman *et al.* 1996, Cookson *et al.* 1998). This may, however, have been related to incorrect handling of these devices (Do *et al.* 1999). Recent clinical trials have shown that these devices need to be carefully decontaminated particularly after drawing blood through them. Indeed, the connectors need to be cleaned with antiseptic both before and after withdrawing or giving blood through them. If this is carried out, the risk of infection may be reduced as compared to standard luer devices (Seymour *et al.* 2000, Casey *et al.* 2003, 2007).

Antimicrobial lock solution

Another approach to prevent catheter-related sepsis has been the installation of an antimicrobial solution into the catheter lumen. The antimicrobial remains locked in situ usually for up to 12 hours in the internal lumen of the catheter. This technique has been shown to be mainly effective for the prevention of infection with long-term CVCs (Shwartz *et al.* 1990, Rackoff *et al.* 1995). This approach has, however, not had universal acceptance as a technique for the prevention of catheter-related sepsis as it may increase antimicrobial resistance. Antimicrobial locks have been more widely used as part of therapy for these infections (Elliott 2004).

Prophylactic thrombolysis

The use of an anticoagulant agent, for example heparin, has been shown to reduce the incidence of catheter thrombosis (Rackoff *et al.* 1995) and subsequent sepsis. This approach reduces the amount of deposited fibronectin on the catheter surface which facilitates the attachment of staphylococci. In a meta-analysis evaluating the benefit of heparin prophylaxis, the risk of catheter-related thrombosis was reduced (Randolph *et al.* 1998a). There was also a significant decrease in bacterial colonisation of the catheters and an associated reduction in bloodstream infections with the use of heparin. This strategy, however, requires further evaluation to fully determine the value of anticoagulants for this purpose.

In-line filters

Studies have demonstrated that the use of 0.22 μm filters incorporated into giving sets reduces the risk of phlebitis (Falchuk *et al.* 1985). There are, however, no adequate studies which demonstrate that filters reduce the risk of catheter-related infections, and they are therefore not routinely recommended currently for prevention (Mermel 2000).

The patient

Most aspects of patient care associated with the insertion, use and subsequent mainte-nance of the catheter are important in the prevention of related infections. The main factors which need to be considered in any preventative strategy are presented below.

Site of insertion

Insertion of CVC into the femoral vein is associated with a higher risk of infection than those inserted into the internal jugular (Lorente *et al.* 2008). Prospective observational studies using multi-variant analysis have demonstrated that the risk of infection was significantly increased with insertion of catheters into the internal jugular as compared to the subclavian vein (Mermel *et al.* 1991, Mermel 2000). Insertion of a catheter into the subclavian vein may therefore reduce the risk of an infection. The choice of insertion site, however, also needs to be balanced with other risk factors associated with this procedure.

Subcutaneous tunnelling

Subcutaneous tunnelling of short-term catheters inserted into the internal jugular vein reduced the risk of catheter-related infections (Timsit *et al.* 1996). In comparison, sub-cutaneous tunnelling of subclavian vein catheters did not significantly reduce the risk of associated septicaemia (Randolph *et al.* 1998b). Tunnelling of short-term CVC is not currently recommended.

Disinfection of the insertion site

Thorough cleansing and disinfection of the skin site of insertion are essential. Disinfec-tion of intravascular catheter insertion sites with 2% aqueous chlorhexidine reduces the associated infection rate as compared to the use of 10% povidone-iodine and 70% alcohol (Maki *et al.* 1991). In comparison, preparations with lower concentration of chlorhexidine are not as effective. For example 0.5% chlorhexidine gluconate has been shown not to be as effective as 10% povidone-iodine (Humar *et al.* 2000). These results have been supported recently by evidence from our group that 2% chlorhexidine in 70% alcohol is more effective at killing organisms in biofilms and in the presence of protein (Adams *et al.* 2005) than a range of other commonly used antiseptics. Chlorhexidine exhibits broad-spectrum antimicrobial activity against the common skin commensals which can cause catheter-related infections. However, 2% chlorhexidine with 70% isopropyl alcohol is now commercially available. Alcoholic chlorhexidine is now rec-ommended as a skin preparation prior to CVC insertion (Pratt *et al.* 2007).

Dressings

The risk of patients developing CVC-related bloodstream infections has been shown to be similar for both transparent and gauze dressings when applied to the site of insertion

(Hoffman *et al.* 1992, Maki 1995). Other conflicting reports have suggested that the use of either gauze or permeable transparent dressings may result in a reduction of sepsis rates (Baranowski 1989, Reynolds *et al.* 1997, Do *et al.* 1999). These reports suggest that the choice of CVC dressings is still open to debate. It would, however, seem a logical approach to initially use a gauze dressing if blood or other serous fluid is oozing from the catheter insertion site (Maki and Will 1984) which can occur particularly during the first 48 hours following catheter insertion. If a transparent dressing has an acceptable water vapour transfer factor which also allows direct observation of the insertion site on a regular basis, as part of appropriate catheter care, their use when the wound no longer oozes fluid seems a logical approach.

Antimicrobial ointments around catheter insertion site

Several randomised studies have investigated the efficacy of various antibiotic ointments applied to the insertion site once the catheter has been inserted. The results, however, have been relatively unclear primarily because of the low numbers of infections in the reported trials (Maki and Band 1981). Interestingly, the application of a mupirocin ointment to the insertion site of dialysis catheters has been shown to reduce the risk of catheter-related bloodstream infections with *S. aureus* (Sesso *et al.* 1998). Conversely, mupirocin resistance may ensue. Mupirocin can also interact with polyurethane catheter material changing its composition and function (Riu *et al.* 1998). In comparison, the role of povidone-iodine ointment applied to the catheter exit site is still unclear (Maki and Will 1986). However, when povidone-iodine was applied to haemodialysis catheter insertion sites, it reduced the incidence of exit site infections (Levin *et al.* 1991).

Catheter replacement and/or guide by exchange

Increased duration of catheterisation has been linked to an increased risk of catheter-related infections (Safdar *et al.* 2004). However, in a controlled study replacing catheters on a routine basis rather than on detection of sepsis failed to show a reduction in risk (Cobb *et al.* 1992). Guidewire exchange may also increase the risk of infection of the new catheter. However, randomised prospective studies have not detected any preventative benefit associated with guidewire exchange compared to insertion at a new site (Badley *et al.* 1996). Guidewire exchange with microbiological culture of the explanted catheter tip is essential in patients when sepsis is suspected without clinical evidence of other sources of infection (Eggimann *et al.* 2000). If the explanted catheter is subsequently shown to be colonised and possibly a source of sepsis then removal of the new device can take place and another device inserted at a new site.

Health care workers

Hand hygiene methods

Infection control is essential in applying aseptic techniques to prevent catheter-related infections. This includes the application of standard infection control precautions, the strict adherence to washing of hands and skin disinfection when caring for patients including devices (Larson 1995). Compliance with hand hygiene has been reported to be relatively low (Sproat and Inglis 1994). Eggimann *et al.* (2000), however, recently demonstrated that the use of simple bedside hand disinfection techniques resulted in sustained improvement in compliance with hand hygiene over a 4-year period. It is evident therefore that hand hygiene needs to be simple and readily available if it is to be used on a regular basis (Pittet *et al.* 2000).

Educational programmes

Educational programmes for physicians in training can decrease the risk of catheter-related infections. Eggimann *et al.* (2000) reported the results of a study which evaluated the impact of a global strategy targeted at reducing catheter-related infections in patients admitted to a medical intensive care unit. The programme targeted vascular access care and consisted of staff bedside training. Following the introduction of this programme, both localised infections and bloodstream infections related to catheters were significantly reduced (Eggimann *et al.* 2000). Interestingly, the reduction of nosocomial infections was superior to that from the use of antimicrobial- or antiseptic-coated catheters. The results of such an educational programme supports the contention that specialised trained teams for catheter insertion and care should be considered.

Conclusion

Recommendations

The main recommendations for the prevention of intravascular catheter-related infections are summarised below. These recommendations reflect those in High Impact Intervention 1 of the Saving Lives toolkit (UK DOH).

(1) Device
   - Use a single lumen CVC unless otherwise indicated.
   - Use an antimicrobial CVC if the device is required for between 1 and 3 weeks and risk of catheter-related bloodstream infection is high.
   - Replace administration sets immediately post-blood administration, every 24 h if administering parenteral nutrition and every 72 h for other fluids.
   - Do not routinely replace CVC.
(2) patient
   - Use 2% chlorhexidine gluconate in 70% isopropyl alcohol for skin preparation prior to CVC insertion (povidone-iodine for patients who are allergic to chlorhexidine gluconate).
   - Insert the CVC into a subclavian or jugular vein rather than femoral.
   - Use Sterile, transparent, semi-permeable dressings.
   - Use aseptic technique and swab the CVC hubs or ports with 2% chlorhexidine gluconate in 70% isopropyl alcohol prior to accessing the CVC.
(3) Healthcare worker
   - Full barrier precautions should be used for the insertion of CVC.
   - Decontaminate hands before and after each patient contact using the correct hand hygiene procedure.

- Single use gloves should be worn during catheter accessing or maintenance.
- On a daily basis healthcare workers should inspect CVC exit sites for signs of infection.

Many approaches to the prevention of catheter-related infection have been applied. It is evident that continuous audit of these infections is important to ensure that any unit is aware of their current rates of infection. Such audit is the most critical point of the continuing prevention of these infections.

References

Adams D, Quayum MH, Worthington T *et al.* (2005). Evaluation of a 2% chlorhexidine gluconate in 70% isopropyl alcohol skin disinfectant. *Journal of Hospital Infection* 61:287–290.

Arnow PM, Quimosing EM, Beach M (1993). Consequences of intravascular catheter sepsis. *Clinical Infectious Disease* 16:778–784.

Bach A, Schmidt H, Bottiger B *et al.* (1996). Retention of antibacterial activity and bacterial colonization of antiseptic-bonded central venous catheters. *Journal of Antimicrobial Chemotherapy* 37:315–322.

Badley AD, Steckelberg JM, Wollan PC *et al.* (1996) Infectious rates of central venous pressure catheters: comparison between newly placed catheters and those that have been changed. *Mayo Clinic Proceedings* 71:838–846.

Baranowski L (1989). Central venous access devices; current technologies, uses and management strategies. *Journal of Intravenous Nursing* 126:167–194.

Casey AL, Worthington T, Lambert PA *et al.* (2003). A randomized, prospective clinical trial to assess the potential infection risk associated with the PosiFlow needleless connector. *Journal of Hospital Infection* 54:288–293.

Casey AL, Burnell S, Whinn H *et al.* (2007). A prospective clinical trial to evaluate the microbial barrier of a needless connector. *Journal of Hospital Infection* 65(3):212–218.

Casey AL, Mermel LA, Nightingale P *et al.* (2008). Antimicrobial central venous catheters – where are we now? Review and meta-analyses of devices evaluated in adults. *Lancet Infectious Diseases*, in press.

Chatzinikolaou I, Finkel K, Hanna H *et al.* (2003). Antibiotic-coated hemodialysis catheters for the prevention of vascular catheter-related infections: a prospective randomized study. *American Journal of Medicine* 115:352–357.

Ciresi DL, Albrecht RM, Volkers PA *et al.* (1996). Failure of antiseptic bonding to prevent central venous catheter-related infection and sepsis. *American Surgeon* 62:641–664.

Cobb DK, High KP, Sawyer RG *et al.* (1992). A controlled trial of scheduled replacement of central venous and pulmonary-artery catheters. *New England Journal of Medicine* 327:1062–1068.

Collin GR (1999). Decreasing catheter colonization through the use of an antiseptic-impregnated catheter: a continuous quality improvement project. *Chest* 115:1632–1640.

Cookson ST, Ihrig M, O'Mara EM *et al.* (1998). Increased bloodstream infection rates in surgical patients associated with variation from recommended use and care following implementation of a needleless device. *Infection Control Hospital Epidemiology* 19:28–31.

Darouiche RO, Raad II, Heard SO *et al.* (1999). A comparison of two antimicrobial-impregnated central venous catheters. *New England Journal of Medicine* 340:1–8.

Do AN, Ray BJ, Banerjee SN *et al.* (1999). Bloodstream infection associated with needleless devices use and the importance of infection control practices in the home health care setting. *Journal of Infectious Diseases* 179:442–448.

Dunser MW, Mayr AJ, Hinterberger G *et al.* (2005). Central venous catheter colonization in critically ill patients: a prospective, randomized, controlled study comparing standard with two antiseptic-impregnated catheters. *Anesthesia and Analgesia* 101:1778-1784.

Eggimann P, Harbarth S, Constantin MN *et al.* (2000). Impact of a prevention strategy targeted at vascular-access care on incidence of infections acquired in intensive care. *Lancet* 355:1864–1868.

Eggimann P, Pittet D (2002). Overview of catheter-related infections with special emphasis on prevention based on education programs. *Clinical Microbiology Infection* 8:295–309.

Elliott TSJ (1988). Intravascular-device infections. *Journal of Medical Microbiology* 27:161–167.

Elliott TSJ (1997). Catheter-associated infections: new developments in prevention. In *Current Topics in Intensive Care*, Buchard H (ed.), Vol. 4. WB Saunders, London, pp. 182–205.

Elliott TSJ (1999a). Can antimicrobial central venous catheters prevent associated infection? *British Journal of Haematology* 107:235–241.

Elliott TSJ (1999b). Role of antimicrobial central venous catheters for the prevention of associated infections. *Journal of Antimicrobial Chemotherapy* 43:441–446.

Elliott TSJ (2000). Intravascular catheter-related sepsis-novel methods of prevention. *Intensive Care Medicine* 26:S45–S50.

Elliott TSJ (2001). The prevention of central venous catheter-related sepsis. *Journal of Chemotherapy* 13:234–238.

Elliott TSJ (2004). The management and treatment of intravascular catheter-related infections. In *Catheter-Related Infections in the Critically Ill*, O'Grady PN, Pittet D (eds), Vol. 8, Springer, USA, pp. 113–126.

Falchuk KH, Peterson L, McNeil BJ (1985). Microparticulate-induced phlebitis. Its prevention by in-line filtration. *New England Journal of Medicine* 312:78–82.

Hanna H, Benjamin R, Chatzinikolaou I *et al.* (2004). Long-term silicone central venous catheters impregnated with minocycline and rifampin decrease rates of catheter-related bloodstream infection in cancer patients: a prospective randomized clinical trial. *Journal of Clinical Oncology* 22:3163–3171 (erratum: *J Clin Oncol* 2005;23:3652).

Hannan M, Juste RN, Umasanker S *et al.* (1999). Antiseptic-bonded central venous catheters and bacterial colonization. *Anaesthesia* 54:868–872.

Heard SO, Wagle M, Vijayakumar E *et al.* (1998). Influence of triple-lumen central venous catheters coated with chlorhexidine and silver sulfadiazine on the incidence of catheter-related bacteremia. *Archives of Internal Medicine* 158:81–78.

Henderson DK (1988). Intravascular device associated infection: current concepts and controversies. *Infection and Surgery* 4:365–400.

Hoffman KK, Weber DJ, Samsa GP *et al.* (1992). Transparent polyurethane film as an intravenous catheter dressing. A meta-analysis of the infection risks. *JAMA* 267:2072–2076.

Humar A, Ostromecki A, Direnfeld J *et al.* (2000). Prospective randomised trial of 10% povidone iodine versus 0.5% tincture of chlorhexidine as cutaneous antisepsis with central venous catheter infections. *Clinical Infectious Disease* 31:1001–1007.

Jaeger K, Zenz S, Juttner B *et al.* (2005). Reduction of catheter-related infections in neutropenic patients: a prospective controlled randomized trial using a chlorhexidine and silver sulfadiazine-impregnated central venous catheter. *Annals of Hematology* 84:258–262.

Kellerman S, Shay DK, Howard J *et al.* (1996). Bloodstream infections in home infusion patients: the influence of race and needleless intravascular devices. *Journal of Pediatrics* 129:711–717.

Larson EL (1995). APIC guidelines for handwashing and hand antisepsis in health care settings. *American Journal of Infection Control* 23:251–269.

Leon C, Ruiz-Santana S, Rello J *et al.* (2004). Benefits of minocycline and rifampin-impregnated central venous catheters. A prospective, randomized, double-blind, controlled, multicenter trial. *Intensive Care Medicine* 30:1891–1899.

Levin A, Mason AJ, Jindal KK *et al.* (1991). Prevention of hemodialysis subclavian vein catheter infections by topical povidone-iodine. *Kidney International* 40:934–938.

Linares J, Sitges-Serra A, Garau J *et al.* (1985). Pathogenesis of catheter sepsis: a prospective study with quantitative and semiquantitative cultures of catheter hub and segments. *Journal of clinical Microbiology* 21(3):357–360.

Logghe C, Van Ossel C, D'Hoore W *et al.* (1997). Evaluation of chlorhexidine and silver-sulfadiazine impregnated central venous catheters for the prevention of bloodstream infection in leukaemic patients: a randomized controlled trial. *Journal of Hospital Infection* 37:145–156.

Lorente L, Jimenez A, Garcia C *et al.* (2008). Catheter-related bacteremia from femoral and central internal jugular venous access. *European Journal of Clinical Microbiology and Infectious Diseases* 27(9):867–871.

Luna J, Masdeu G, Perez M *et al.* (2000) Clinical trial evaluating a new hub device designate to prevent catheter-related sepsis. *European Journal of Clinical Microbiology and Infectious Diseases* 19:655–662.

Maki DG (1992) Infections due to infusion therapy. In *Hospital Infections*, Maki DG, Brachman PS, Bennett JV (eds), 3rd edn. Little Brown, Boston, pp. 849–898.

Maki DG, Band JD (1981). A comparative study of polyantibiotic and iodophor ointments in prevention of vascular catheter-related infection. *American Journal of Medicine* 70:739–744.

Maki DG, Ringer M, Alvarado CJ (1991). Prospective randomised trial of povidone-iodine, alcohol and chlorhexidine for prevention of infection associated with central venous and arterial catheters. *Lancet* 338:339–343.

Maki DG, Stolz S, Wheeler S *et al.* (1994). A prospective randomized trial of gauze and two polyurethane dressings for site care of pulmonary artery catheters: implications for catheter management. *Critical Care Medicine* 22:1729–1737.

Maki DG, Will L (1984). Colonization and infection associated with transparent dressing for central venous, arterial and Hickman catheters: a comparative trial (Abstract). In *Programs and Abstracts of the 24th Interscience Conference on Antimicrobial Agents and Chemotherapy*, 8–10 October 1984, Washington DC. *American Society for Microbiology*, 230.

Maki DG, Will L (1986). Study of polyantibiotic and povidone-iodine ointments on central venous and arterial catheter sites dressed with gauze or polyurethane dressing (Abstract). In *Programs and Abstracts of the 26th Interscience Conference on Antimicrobial Agents and Chemotherapy*, 28 September–1 October 1986, New Orleans, Louisiana, Washington DC. *American Society for Microbiology*, 1041.

Maki DG, Stolz SS, Wheeler S, Mermel LA (1994). A prospective, randomized trial of gauze and two polyurethane dressings for site care of pulmonary artery catheters: implications for catheter management. *Critical Care Medicine* 22(11):1729–1237.

Maki DG, Stolz SM, Wheeler S *et al.* (1997). Prevention of central venous catheter-related bloodstream infection by use of an antiseptic-impregnated catheter. A randomized, controlled trial. *Annals of Internal Medicine* 127:257–266.

Marciante KD, Veenstra DL, Lipsky BA *et al.* (2003). Which antimicrobial impregnated catheters should be used? Modelling the costs and outcome of antimicrobial catheter use. *American Journal of Infection Control* 31:128.

Marik PE, Abraham G, Careau P *et al.* (1999). The *ex vivo* antimicrobial activity and colonization rate of two antimicrobial-bonded central venous catheters. *Critical Care Medicine* 27:1128–1131.

Mermel LA (2000). Prevention of intravascular catheter-related infections. *Annuals of Internal Medicine* 132:391–402.

Mermel LA, McCormick RD, Springman SR *et al.* (1991). The pathogenesis and epidemiology of catheter-related infection with pulmonary artery Swan-Ganz catheters a prospective study utilizing molecular subtyping. *American Journal of Medicine* 3B:197S–205S.

Oda T, Hamasaki J, Kanda N *et al.* (1997). Anaphylactic shock induced by an antiseptic coated central venous catheter. *Anaesthesiology* 87:1242–1244.

Osma S, Kahveci SF, Kaya FN *et al.* (2006). Efficacy of antiseptic-impregnated catheters on catheter colonization and catheter-related bloodstream infections in patients in an intensive care unit. *Journal of Hospital Infection* 62:156–162.

Pearson ML (1996). Guideline for prevention of intravascular device-related infections. Hospital infection control practices advisory committee. *Infection Control Hospital Epidemiology* 17:438–473.

Pemberton LB, Ross V, Cuddy P *et al.* (1996). No difference in catheter sepsis between standard and antiseptic central venous catheters. A prospective randomized trial. *Archives of Surgery* 131:986–989.

Pittet D, Hugonnet S, Harbarth S *et al.* (2000). Effectiveness of a hospital-wide programme to improve compliance with hand hygiene. *Lancet* 356:1307–1312.

Pittet D, Hulliger S, Auckenthaler R (1995). Intravascular device-related infections in critically ill patients. *Journal of Chemotherapy* 7:55–66.

Pratt RJ, Pellowe CM, Wilson JA *et al.* (2007). Epic 2: National-Evidence Based Guidelines for Preventing Healthcare-Associated Infections in NHS Hospitals in England. Department of Health (England). *Journal of Hospital Infection* 65(Suppl 1):S1–S64.

Raad I, Darouiche R, Dupuis J *et al.* (1997). Central venous catheters coated with minocycline and rifampicin for the prevention of catheter-related colonization and bloodstream infections. A randomized double-blind trial. The Texas Medical Center Catheter Study Group. *Annuals of Internal Medicine* 127:267–274.

Rackoff WR, Weiman M, Jakobowski D *et al.* (1995). A randomized controlled trial of the efficacy of a heparin and vancomycin solution in preventing central venous catheter infection in children. *Journal of Pediatrics* 127:147–151.

Randolph AG, Cook DJ, Gonzales CA *et al.* (1998a). Benefit of heparin in central venous and pulmonary artery catheters: a meta-analysis of randomised controlled trials. *Chest* 113:165–171.

Randolph AG, Cook DJ, Gonzales CA *et al.* (1998b). Tunneling short-term central venous catheters to prevent catheter-related infection: a meta-analysis of randomized, controlled trials. *Critical Care Medicine* 26:1452–1457.

Reynolds MG, Tebbs SE, Elliott TSJ (1997). Do dressings with increased permeability reduce the incidence of central venous catheter related sepsis? *Intensive Critical Care Nursing* 13:26–29.

Riu S, Ruiz CG, Martinez-Vera A *et al.* (1998). Spontaneous rupture of polyurethane peritoneal catheter. A possible deleterious effect of mupirocin ointment. *Nephrology Dialysis Transplantation* 13:1870–1871.

Safdar N, Mermel L, Maki DG (2004). The epidemiology of catheter-related infection in the critically ill. *Catheter-Related Infections in the Critically Ill*, O'Grady PN, Pittet D (eds), Vol. 8, Springer, New York, USA, 1–22.

Salzman MB, Isenberg HD, Shapiro JF *et al.* (1993). A prospective study of the catheter hub as the portal of entry for microorganisms causing catheter-related sepsis in neonates. *Journal of Infectious Diseases* 167:487–490.

Segura M, Alvarez-Lerma F, Tellado JM *et al.* (1996). A clinical trial on the prevention of catheter-related sepsis using a new hub model. *Annuals of Surgery* 223:363–369.

Sesso R, Barbosa D, Leme IL *et al.* (1998). *Staphylococcus aureus* prophylaxis in hemodialysis patients using central venous catheter: effect of mupirocin ointment. *Journal of American Society of Nephrology* 9:1085–1092.

Seymour VM, Dhallu TS, Moss HA *et al.* (2000). A prospective clinical study to investigate the microbial contamination of a needleless connector. *Journal of Hospital Infection* 45:165–168.

Shwartz C, Henrickson KJ, Roghmann K *et al.* (1990). Prevention of bacteremia attributed to luminal colonization of tunnelled central venous catheter with vancomycin susceptible organisms. *Journal of Clinical Oncology* 8:591–597.

Sheng WH, Ko WJ, Wang JT *et al.* (2000). Evaluation of antiseptic-impregnated central venous catheters for prevention of catheter-related infection in intensive care unit patients. *Diagnostic Microbiology and Infectious Diseases* 38:1–5.

Sitges-Serra A, Hernandej R, Maestro S *et al.* (1997) Prevention of catheter sepsis: the hub. *Nutrition* 13:305–355.

Sproat LJ, Inglis TJ (1994). A multi-centre survey of hand hygiene practice in intensive care units. *Journal of Hospital Infection* 26:137–148.

Stephens R, Whyson N, Kallis P *et al.* (2001) Two episodes of life threatening anaphylaxis in the patient to chlorhexidine sulphadiazine coated central venous catheter. *British Journal of Anaesthesiology* 87:306–308.

Tebbs SE, Elliott TSJ (1994). Modifications of central venous catheter polymers to prevent in vitro microbial colonisation. *European Journal of Clinical Microbiology and Infection Disease* 13:111–117.

Tebbs SE, Ghose A, Elliott TSJ (1996). Microbial contamination of intravenous and arterial catheters. *Intensive Care Medicine* 22:272–273.

Tennenberg S, Lieser M, McCurdy B *et al.* (1997). A prospective randomized trial of an antibiotic- and antiseptic-coated central venous catheter in the prevention of catheter-related infections. *Archives of Surgery* 132:1348–1351.

Timsit JF, Sebille V, Farkas JC *et al.* (1996). Effect of subcutaneous tunneling on internal jugular catheter-related sepsis in critically ill patients. A prospective randomized multicenter study. *JAMA* 276:1415–1420.

Trim JC, Elliott TSJ (2003). A review of sharps injuries and preventative strategies. *Journal of Hospital Infection* 53:237–242.

UK DOH. The recent Savings lives document. http://www.dh.gov.uk/en/Publichealth/Healthprotection/Healthcareacquiredinfection/ Healthcareacquired generalinformation/Thedeliveryprogrammetoreducehealthcareassociated infectionsHCAIincludingMRSA/index.htm

van Heerden PV, Webb SA, Fong S *et al.* (1996). Central venous catheters revisited-infection rates and an assessment of the new Fibrin Analysing System brush. *Anaesthesia and Intensive Care* 24:330–333.

Worthington T, Elliott TSJ (2005). Diagnosis of central venous catheter related infection in adult patients. *Journal of Infection* 51:267–280.

Chapter 14

Aftercare and management of central venous access devices

Liz Bishop

Introduction

Great emphasis is placed on the safe insertion of central vascular access devices (CVADs); however, the aftercare must be of equally high standard if device-related morbidity and mortality are to be kept to a minimum and if the catheter is to remain working for the required length of time. The care and management of CVADs should be evidence-based where possible and suited to the type and site of the device.

In the clinical setting, there is a wide variation of practice and opinion, which can further contribute to confusion. To further complicate matters, the devices themselves and aids to safely manage them are constantly changing. The purpose of this chapter is to provide a comprehensive standard of care for CVADs based on the most recent available evidence. It is important that health care professionals who care for CVADs are familiar with and knowledgeable on the devices used in their particular clinical area, otherwise complications will occur. For example, using the wrong flushing solution may lead to catheter occlusion or the wrong size of syringe may lead to catheter rupture. Ideally, any comprehensive vascular access service should not only include an insertion service but an aftercare education programme and advisory/consultancy service or directly provide the aftercare as part of the service. Locally developed guidelines for the insertion, care and management of CVADs may also assist in the reducing complications post-insertion.

Learning outcomes are:

- To understand the principles of minimising/reducing CVAD infection rates
- To understand the principles of preventing catheter occlusion and maintaining device integrity
- To understand the principles of preventing catheter-related thrombosis

Immediate patient care post-catheter insertion

The patient should be recovered depending on what level of anaesthesia and sedation has been used and according to local protocol. Sedation and anaesthesia can cause respiratory depression and alterations in the cardiovascular system, therefore pulse oximetry and assessment of pulse, respiration rate and blood pressure are required during and post-procedure until the patient is awake and alert (Craig 2003).

Although fluoroscopic-guided device insertion provides information about tip position, the resultant small focused images are difficult for later interpretation, particularly for inexperienced staff. It is recommended that tip placement should be checked and documented by an upright chest X-ray prior to use, to exclude pneumothorax and other complications (RCN 2005). Optimal tip position is the lower third of the superior vena cava or upper right atrium (Fletcher and Bodenham 2000). If the catheter tip resides in the upper right atrium, this is acceptable if there are no associated arrhythmias. A further chest X-ray is required if the patient becomes dyspnoeic or develops a cough or shoulder tip pain as there is a 1–2% incidence of pneumothorax post-operatively, which can occur several hours later (Ray *et al.* 1996). Some centres wait for 2 hours following device insertion for the chest X-ray to exclude pneumothorax for this reason. The issue of pneumothorax is covered in detail in Chapter 12.

After the procedure, the dressing should be changed if bleeding has occurred, but otherwise, not changed until 24–48 hours post-operatively (RCN 2005). The exit site should be inspected before the patient is discharged home and if necessary the dressing changed. If the patient is to remain in hospital, the exit site should be inspected post-operatively and at a minimum of daily thereafter (RCN 2005), with any changes documented or reported as per local policy. If the patient is thrombocytopenic and there is evidence of bleeding post-catheter insertion, the patient should receive further platelet transfusion(s) to maintain the count in excess of $50 \times 10^9 \, L^{-1}$, until the bleeding stops bearing in mind problems may exist in patients (Slichter-Sherrill 2007). In these situations, and in patients with platelet antibodies, application of pressure dressings and topical tranexamic acid may help. In those patients with *disseminated intravascular coagulation*, there should be vigorous correction of any abnormality of coagulation. The prothrombin time should be <1.3 times normal and fibrinogen >1.0 g L^{-1} and haematology advice should be sought. Bleeding via the exit site may be stopped by a fine purse string suture around the wound.

Following PICC (peripherally inserted central catheter) insertion, some centres recommend minimal movement, keeping the arm warm and advising the patient to be well hydrated to avoid mechanical phlebitis (see Chapters 8 and 12). In theory, this will minimise catheter movement as well as minimising intraluminal irritation and this may help prevent mechanical phlebitis, infection and/or thrombosis.

Going home with a CVAD

Locally generated patient information leaflets are recommended, but this is not a substitute for careful and detailed explanation by a health care professional experienced in the care of central venous catheters. Information should be provided with 24-hour cover arrangements to provide a contact for any of the following problems:

- The exit site is red, sore or oozing pus or there is a fever of >38°C
- The catheter becomes damaged or leaks
- The arm becomes swollen or there are enlarged veins on the chest or neck
- Breathlessness or any pain

Long-term care of CVADs

Prevention of catheter-related infection (see also Chapters 12 and 13)

Introduction

Historically, it was believed that catheter-related bloodstream infections (CRBSIs) arose from microbial colonisation at the exit site and external surfaces of the catheter, known as 'microbial tracking' (Figure 14.1). More recently, intraluminal contamination has been implicated as an equally or more important aetiological factor, particularly for long-term applications. This is where organisms are introduced into the hub via contaminated hands of health care personnel (Linares *et al.* 1985) or some other contaminated source. The organisms migrate along the internal surface of the catheter leading to luminal colonisation and bloodstream infection. This is known as the 'hub hypothesis' (Fletcher and Bodenham 1999) and has been indicated in studies where accessing the hub is more frequent and in studies where blood withdrawal occurs via the hub (Groeger *et al.* 1993, Castagnola *et al.* 2003). Handling of the catheter has to be undertaken by experienced and trained personnel (Vanherweghem *et al.* 1986) and implementation of strict aseptic procedures when manipulating the catheter can reduce the risk of infection significantly (Beathard 2003). Studies have shown that specialist teams can reduce infection rates (Hamilton 2004) and where possible such teams should be developed.

Both microbial tracking and hub contamination are implicated in the development of CRBSIs and it is known that the longer the catheter is in situ the more likely it is to become infected (Waghorn 1994). Raad *et al.* (1994) demonstrated hub contamination was the more likely mechanism of infection for long-term catheters (>30 days in situ), whereas skin contamination was the more likely mechanism for short-term catheters (<10 days in situ). Although much less common, studies have also demonstrated a third means of catheter colonisation, that of haematogenous seeding of endogenous bacteria, usually Gram-negative enteric bacilli, whereby normal gut flora migrate to the catheter and colonise the catheter (Groeger *et al.* 1993). These may subsequently flourish and increase in numbers sufficient enough to cause a septicaemia. This may be more important in the immune-compromised patient.

Exit site and general care

Effective handwashing, and the use of a consistent and effective aseptic technique whenever the CVAD is accessed and during procedures involving exit sites, is important

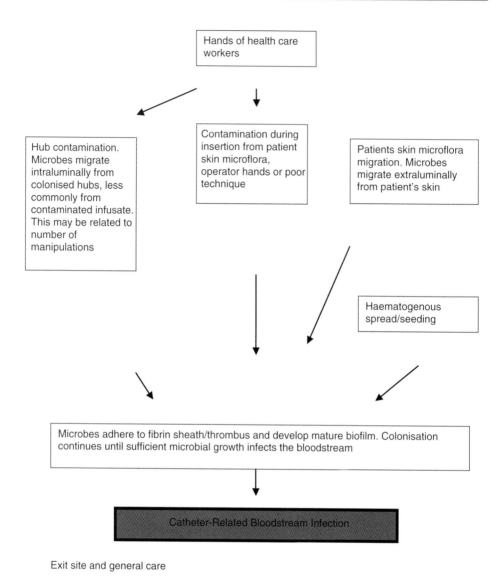

Figure 14.1 Potential sources of contamination in central venous catheters.

(Rowley 1997). Gloves should be worn by nursing staff not only to protect themselves but also to prevent transfer of bacteria onto key parts. Whether or not the gloves should be sterile will depend on the task. For example, accessing the catheter need not require sterile gloves as long as a no-touch technique is used, whereas sterile gloves may be advisable if saline-soaked gauze is used to clean the exit site and handled by the nurse.

It is hard to find convincing research to support any particular exit site cleaning regime. Recent expert opinion favours the use of 2% chlorhexidine gluconate at dressing changes (NICE 2003, RCN 2005, Pratt *et al.* 2007). In the past, use of antiseptics raised concerns amongst some microbiologists, because chlorhexidine was only commercially available in the UK as a relatively weak solution, presented in 500-mL bottles, leading to questions about sterility and resistance. The fact that a sterile single-use preparation of chlorhexidine gluconate 2% in 70% isopropyl alcohol has now become available in the UK may lead to a greater consensus.

Considerable controversy and conflicting evidence surround the issue of what constitutes an ideal exit site dressing and change of dressing regime (Wickham *et al.* 1992, Cornock 1996). The insertion site should be inspected daily for any signs of discomfort or infection (RCN 2005). It should be renewed immediately should it become soiled, wet or detached since a moist environment is one in which bacteria readily multiply. The most suitable dressing will depend on the setting, the type of catheter and the individual patient's needs. Implanted ports do not require any dressing once the wound has healed. PICCs and non-tunnelled catheters should always have a dressing to avoid dislodgement; however, skin-tunnelled catheters with an adequately anchored cuff may not require a dressing (Morris *et al.* 1995). This can be reviewed on an individual basis.

Options for dressings

IV-dedicated occlusive transparent dressing

This dressing has the advantage of allowing continuous inspection of the exit site, and some researchers have found it to be associated with a lower risk of infection than other transparent dressings (Maki and Ringer 1987, Reynolds *et al.* 1997, Treston-Aurend 1997, RCN 2005). Most guidelines suggest that transparent dressings should be changed every 7 days, when fluid is seen to gather beneath the dressing, when the dressing ceases to be occlusive, or whichever is the sooner (RCN 2005). The schedule for the changing of transparent semi-permeable dressings is complex and will depend on the patient's skin, dressing integrity, local infection rates, organisational policy and manufacturer's guidelines, but they should not remain in place longer than 7 days (CDC 2002, NICE 2003, RCN 2005).

Gauze and tape dressing

Sterile dry gauze dressing and tape should be changed every 24 hours (in order that the site may be observed), or whenever the dressing becomes soiled, wet or detached, or whichever occurs sooner (INS 2000, RCN 2005).

No dressing

This may be suitable for some patients with tunnelled CVADs from 21 days post-insertion once the tissues have fibrosed around the cuff and in the absence of exudate or signs of infection (Olson *et al.* 2004). 'No dressing' performed just as well as three types of dressing in one study comparing infection rates (Haller and Rush 1992).

In summary, whatever the dressing, strict asepsis is recommended for dressing changes, irrespective of whether it is unit policy to use sterile gauze and tape or semi-occlusive dressing, the latter having the advantage of allowing visual inspection of the insertion site. However, it does not negate the need for removal of the dressing at established intervals to clean and inspect the site (Dougherty and Lister 2004) particularly if infection is suspected.

Recent expert opinion favours the use of 2% chlorhexidine gluconate at dressing changes (NICE 2003, RCN 2005). The chlorhexidine solution should be liberally applied to the catheter and the area around the catheter and should actually be in contact with the skin for at least 30 seconds. Firm to and fro strokes should be used. The area must then be allowed to air dry completely before a dressing is applied. Similar techniques should be used before accessing a port. After cleaning the skin the access needle is inserted and a semi-occlusive dressing applied.

Keeping the area dry and avoiding bathing/showering is more controversial. Most units allow patients to shower/bathe, but attempt to keep the exit site dry by using occlusive dressing or bathing without submersion of the exit site. Swimming is generally not recommended with any external catheter to prevent colonisation by Gram-negative organisms, especially *Pseudomonas* spp., but a local policy should be developed.

Suture removal

For patients with a skin-tunnelled catheter, the suture over the insertion site incision into the vein may be removed at 7–10 days. The suture at the exit incision and those anchoring the catheter to the skin are important to avoid the cuff exiting the tract and may be removed after about 3 weeks. More recent evidence suggests the routine use of securing devices (e.g. Statlocks, see Chapter 4), particularly with non-tunnelled catheters and PICCs, which negate the need for sutures to attach an anchoring wing near the exit site. These have been shown to reduce infection rates when compared with sutures (Crnich and Maki 2002, Yamamoto 2002, Schears 2005). Sutures over an implanted port insertion site are removed at 7–10 days. Some operators may use absorbable sutures or surgical glue to close all wounds.

Accessing the CVAD

Mermel (2000) in a review described how excessive manipulation of the catheter independently increased the risk of CRBSI, presumably because of greater risk for breaching aseptic technique and increased contamination. Therefore, the number of times a catheter is accessed should be kept to a minimum. There has also been recent emphasis on the need to reduce sharps injuries, which has led to the widespread use of needle-free systems for capping off CVADs. Various conflicting studies have suggested that these devices either increase or decrease CRBSI rates (Tebbs *et al.* 1995). The CDC (2002) examined the available literature and concluded that 'When the devices are used according to manufacturers' recommendations, they do not substantially affect the incidence of CRBSI'. When accessing the catheter, the external surfaces of the hub should be disinfected with a chlorhexidine gluconate solution unless contraindicated by the manufacturer's instructions, immediately prior to access (Pratt *et al.* 2001, NICE 2003, Pellowe *et al.* 2004, RCN 2005). If the needle-free connector is removed from a CVAD, it should be discarded and a new connector attached. The optimal changing times are not known, therefore they must be changed in accordance with manufacturer's recommendations (MHRA 2005, RCN 2005).

Other practices have been recommended to reduce hub contamination. It is recommended that administration sets are changed every 72 hours when used for continuous infusions of solutions, but should be changed more frequently if used for intermittent therapies, or lipids and if there is a breach in the administration set (NICE 2003, RCN 2005). If blood is being infused, the administration set should be changed every 12 hours and a new giving set should be used following transfusion (McClelland 2007, RCN 2005). An aseptic technique should be used to change any giving set.

Flushing solutions

There is a strong link between infection and thrombus, which suggests that reducing thrombus rates should produce a concomitant reduction in infection rates, hence the rationale for using heparin flushes. However, the recent update on guidelines for reducing infections states the 'efficacy of using anticoagulants for preventing CRBSI remains controversial' (Pellowe *et al.* 2004). The Hospital Infection Control Practices Advisory Committee (Pearson 1996) reviewed all the evidence for anticoagulant prophylaxis and concluded that no data demonstrated their use reduced the incidence of CRBSIs and did not recommend them. However, they may be used as prophylaxis for venous thrombosis in those with risk factors, and many clinicians still recommend their use, primarily to maintain catheter patency. It is proposed that systemic antimicrobials do not prevent intraluminal infection; therefore, the use of prophylactic antibiotics is no longer recommended (Pellowe *et al.* 2004, Pratt *et al.* 2007) as the drugs do not reach the internal surface of the catheter. Instead, the technique of 'locking' the catheter with an antimicrobial solution may offer better protection to the inner surface of the device from infection, and in fact many centres use this 'antibiotic lock' technique to treat bloodstream infections. Further details on infection issues are given in Chapter 13.

Maintaining device patency

Patency impairment

Definition and causes

A properly functioning CVC should be easy to flush and allow blood to be withdrawn. Signs and causes of impaired patency are shown in Boxes 14.1 and 14.2.

Box 14.1 Signs of catheter patency impairment.

- The catheter flushes easily but aspiration of blood is sluggish or absent.
- The catheter can be flushed using a syringe but there is sluggish, absent or intermittent free-flow when infusion of fluids by gravity is attempted.
- The catheter is completely blocked and cannot be flushed.

Box 14.2 Other causes of catheter patency impairment.

- Mechanical obstruction: external (e.g. the catheter is kinked or obstructed by a bra-strap or an over-tight stitch); internal (e.g. the catheter is incorrectly positioned and is either kinked or abuts a vessel wall).
- Clotted blood within the catheter due to ineffective flushing techniques.
- Fibrin sheath.
- Vein is completely or partially thrombosed.
- Build up of lipids from TPN or drug precipitation within the catheter. This may be caused by high concentration or incompatibility of drugs.
- Misplacement of catheter in the arterial tree, or other extravascular sites.

A fibrin sheath results from the formation of a thrombus around the catheter within the vein (Teichgräber *et al.* 2003). This gradually transforms into a fibrous collagen substance which may extend from the point at which the catheter enters the vein to the tip of the catheter (Andris *et al.* 1999). Fibrin sheaths are thought to occur in most catheters left in place for over 7 days (Wickham *et al.* 1992, Mayo and Pearson 1995). They may go unnoticed or may impair the patency of the catheter. In severe cases, they may also lead to backtracking of infused fluids between the fibrin sheath and the catheter, causing leakage of those fluids into the tissues (Mayo and Pearson 1995) (see Chapter 10). Fibrin sheaths are associated with an increased risk of infection (Mehall *et al.* 2002) as they provide an ideal medium for the proliferation of bacteria.

Prevention

Correct positioning of the CVC during insertion and proper fixation to prevent dislodgment are vital in ensuring optimum function. Once the CVC is in situ, the focus is on flushing regimes to maintain patency.

Managing impaired patency

Teichgräber *et al.* (2003) states that 'if a CVC device is malfunctioning or is not patent it can be assumed that a complication is present'. Patency problems should be taken seriously, and action taken sooner rather than later to restore full patency. Ignoring the early signs may lead to the development of more serious problems which cannot then be easily rectified – e.g. complete blockage or thrombosis (Hadaway 1998).

Thrombolytics such as urokinase or alteplase are probably the most useful tools in managing impaired patency. Prepared according to the manufacturer's instructions and instilled into the catheter so as to just fill it, they can be locked in place for an hour or two and will often restore the catheter to full function. The dosage is much less than that used for systemic thrombolysis, but nevertheless thrombolytics must be used with caution in patients with impaired coagulation.

In a completely blocked CVC, the temptation to apply a forceful flush using a small syringe must be resisted as this presents a high risk of rupturing the catheter. It is far safer to instil the thrombolytic into the catheter using a three-way tap technique described by Krzywda (1999) (Figure 14.2). Here two syringes are attached to the catheter via a

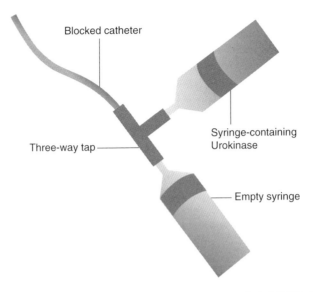

Figure 14.2 Three-way tap technique using two syringes to overcome occluded CVADs (see text for description or technique).

three-way tap – one syringe is empty, the other contains the thrombolytic. The tap is turned to open to the catheter and to the empty syringe, and a vacuum is created in the catheter by pulling back on the plunger. The tap is then turned to open to the second syringe, whereupon the thrombolytic is sucked into the catheter. Catheter clamps should be left open to allow the thrombolytic to mix throughout the length of the lumen. The author has found this technique to be successful many times, although the procedure may need to be repeated several times before the catheter becomes unblocked.

If the use of a thrombolytic fails, and if a build-up of lipids from TPN or drug precipitation within the catheter is thought to be a possible cause of occlusion, advice from a pharmacist should be sought as to which agent might dissolve the occlusion.

A catheter whose full function cannot be restored by the above measures should be investigated further. A chest X-ray will help to exclude malposition, and fluoroscopic examination will throw further light on any obstructions to flow. Some catheters are prone to what has been dubbed persistent withdrawal occlusion (PWO) – probably due to fibrin sheath formation. If patency impairment is accompanied by unexplained and abnormal phenomena relating to the CVC such as leakage of blood or fluids from the exit site, or if the patient experiences discomfort during infusion or flushing, the problem should be fully investigated before the catheter is used.

Maintaining device patency is essential if the CVAD is to last for its intended duration. This requires meticulous attention to flushing protocols and prompt action if occlusion due to thrombosis is suspected (see Chapter 12).

Accessing the device

The patency of the device should be checked prior to the administration of any solutions. Many practitioners routinely withdraw blood prior to flushing, but there is no requirement for this except when blood sampling (RCN 2005) or if strong heparin solution (e.g. 1000 U mL^{-1}) has been used to flush the device, for example, in renal dialysis catheters. Withdrawing blood may actually contribute to an increased risk of infection and occlusion (Gabriel *et al.* 2005) and although there is no evidence for this, expert opinion discourages blood withdrawal from central venous access devices where possible (RCN 2005). The volume of flush should be at least twice the intraluminal volume of the catheter including any add-on devices such as the needle-free connectors (RCN 2005) but usually 5–10 mL is used.

Blood sampling

A blood sampling protocol can be developed locally, but must include instruction on the removal of the heparinised dead space (approximately 5 mL) prior to sampling to avoid erroneous results if heparin solution is used to flush the catheter. The exception would be when taking samples from each lumen for blood cultures where the first sample removed (including dead space) will be included in the sample for culture. The volume to be removed before coagulation studies are performed is uncertain with central venous catheters, but for coagulation studies from arterial cannulae it is recommended that six times the dead space volume be removed (Laxson and Titler 1994). Coagulation studies in such circumstances may produce erroneous results, particularly in the case of apheresis or dialysis catheters where stronger heparin solutions have been used and, if any doubt, the sample should be taken from a peripheral vein. The lumen for taking blood drug levels should be identified and the drugs administered through a different lumen. Similar problems may occur with blood glucose measurements if glucose containing flush solutions is inadvertently used.

Flushing solutions

Traditionally, CVADs have been flushed with saline or heparin solutions, the latter of varying strength depending on the catheter type. It is common to use low-dose intermittent heparin flushes to fill the lumens of CVCs between uses, in an attempt to prevent thrombus formation and to prolong the duration of catheter life but the efficacy of this practice is unproven (Pellowe *et al.* 2004, Pratt *et al.* 2007). Therefore, 0.9% saline should be used as standard. The use of heparinised saline may be justified in implanted devices or open-ended devices when the catheter is used infrequently. In implantable ports, less frequent flushing with a higher concentration of heparinised saline (e.g. 100 or 500 U mL^{-1}) tends to be recommended when the port is not in use (Vygon 2000). It is common practice in CVCs designed for haemodialysis or apheresis to lock the catheter with a concentrated solution of heparin (e.g. 1000 U mL^{-1}) which must be withdrawn from the catheter prior to flushing. Other citrate-based solutions are also under study (Lok-Charmaine *et al.* 2007). Here the open-ended design of the catheter – essential for dialysis or apheresis – makes reflux more likely and there is a crucial need to maintain patency. These catheters are generally cared for by specialist personnel aware of the dangers of inadvertently flushing the heparin out of the catheter into the circulation.

Exposure to heparin should be minimised to prevent the development of heparin-induced thrombocytopenia (HIT), which can occur in 2.7% of patients exposed to unfractionated heparin (Warkentin *et al.* 1995), and the potential to develop bleeding complications through inadvertent heparinisation following multiple heparin flushes (Passannante and Macik 1998). Flushing protocols for the main types of catheter are

Table 14.1 Central venous catheter flushing protocols.

Catheter type	Solution	Frequency	Cautions
Non-tunnelled	Saline 0.9% ± Weak heparin solution (10 U mL^{-1})	After each access or at least weekly	
Skin-tunnelled[a]	Saline 0.9% ± Weak heparin solution (10 U mL^{-1})	After each access or at least weekly	
Ports[a]	Saline 0.9% ± Weak heparin solution (10 U mL^{-1})	After each access or at least monthly	No syringe of less than 10 mL size to avoid catheter rupture
Apheresis/dialysis	Saline 0.9% + heparin 1000 U mL^{-1} or 5000 U mL^{-1} *intraluminal volume only*	After each access or at least weekly	Note 'dead space' space volume on catheter to avoid systemic heparinisation
PICCs[a]	Saline 0.9% ± Weak heparin solution (10 U mL^{-1})	After each access or at least weekly	

[a] Valved catheters require 10 mL saline 0.9% solution to flush. No heparin required.

shown in Table 14.1, although one must always refer to the manufacturer's recommendations.

Flushing technique

The technique used to flush the CVAD is also important, for example it is vital the correct syringe size is used (see below). During the flushing process, care must always be taken to maintain patency by using a pulsatile flush method and maintaining positive pressure while removing the syringe at the end of flushing in order to avoid reflux of blood (Goodwin and Carlson 1993, Dougherty and Lister 2004, RCN 2005). It is thought the pulsatile flushing method creates turbulence inside the catheter and may assist with removal of debris on the internal walls of the catheter and reduce the chances of an intraluminal clot (Todd 1998, Gabriel *et al.* 2005, RCN 2005).

Dedicated connectors are available which automatically deliver a small bolus into the catheter when the syringe is disconnected. Alternatively, a positive pressure finish can be achieved by clamping the catheter while the final volume of the flush is being injected. In a valved line which has no clamp, the same effect can be obtained by removing the syringe from the connector while injecting the last millilitre, though it is advisable to wrap gauze around the connector during this procedure in order to avoid any spray from the syringe.

Frequency and volume of flush

In the light of work done by Kelly (1992), the RCN (2005) recommends that:

- Unused lumens should be flushed weekly and only more often if problems arise.

- The flushing solution should be 'at least twice the volume of the catheter and add-on devices, usually 5–10 mL'.
- Saline (0.9%) should be used before, between and after incompatible drugs and solutions to reduce the likelihood of precipitation and drug interactions.

Prevention of catheter-related vein thrombosis

Thrombus formation can occur at any time following insertion of a CVAD. The patient may have undiagnosed thrombophilia related to disease states (e.g. malignancy) and drug therapy (e.g. thalidomide), or it may occur spontaneously. Thrombus may initially present as PWO or an inability to infuse solutions. Resistance may be felt when flushing the device. In the case of PICCs or subclavian catheters, it may be suspected when the arm or the hand swells. In the presence of a subclavian thrombosis, the jugular veins or superficial vessels on the chest wall may appear engorged. Unilateral internal jugular thrombosis often has no clinical signs. The thrombus probably originates at the point where the device enters the vein or where there is intraluminal damage, e.g. where the device irritates the internal lumen of the vein. The thrombus may enlarge and/or migrate along the length of the device and eventually occlude the tip. Blockage of the device may occur and the vein thrombosis may completely or partially occlude major vessels. Pulmonary embolus can be a serious sequel to thrombus formation and can occur in from both upper and lower body sites of central venous access (Heit *et al.* 2002, Cox *et al.* 2003). Such embolic clot may also be infected to cause severe systemic sepsis and lung abscess formation (Cook *et al.* 2005).

The importance of catheter tip position

Increased rates of thrombosis have been demonstrated with sub-optimal tip positions; therefore, correct positioning should be ensured and documented at the time of insertion. There continues to be debate as to which route of access carries the lowest risk of catheter-related thrombosis. Some studies demonstrate lowest risk with the subclavian approach (Timsit *et al.* 1998). However, multiple studies have shown the opposite, concluding that subclavian venous catheterisation results in a much higher incidence of venous stenosis and thrombosis than catheterisation via the internal jugular approach (Cimochowski *et al.* 1990, Macdonald *et al.* 2000, Trerotola *et al.* 2000). There is also debate about left- and right-sided catheters. Such differences may relate in part because clinicians may not optimise catheter tip position and use fixed length catheters which will not be ideal for all sites of access.

Anticoagulation

Intraluminal thrombosis may be prevented by adhering to appropriate flushing protocols as described earlier (see Table 14.1); however, this will have little impact on extraluminal thrombosis. Over the years, it has become common practice to use low-dose warfarin, e.g. 1 mg warfarin daily, which is generally a sub-therapeutic dose, to minimise the risk of thrombosis. Recent evidence, however, suggests that the use of low-dose warfarin is of no apparent benefit for the prophylaxis of symptomatic catheter-related thrombosis in patients with cancer (Couban *et al.* 2005, Akl *et al.* 2007). Some clinicians may still continue to prescribe low-dose warfarin in patients with long-term CVADs in situ. Therapeutic dose warfarin should be superior and some centres now use therapeutic dose low molecular weight heparin (Lee 2005) but at the cost of increased risk of bleeding. Full anticoagulation may be warranted if the patient has had previous thromboembolic events, but decisions need to be individualised for each patient (Akl *et al.* 2007).

Maintaining integrity of the device

Patient education is important in maintaining device integrity, particularly if the patient is going home with the device in situ. Any external device should be well secured, and in the case of cuffed skin-tunnelled varieties, especially for the initial 3 weeks. Tension should not be applied to the external portion of the catheter to avoid catheter dislodgement. PICCs are particularly susceptible to movement, hence the use of securing devices is recommended and care should be taken when removing an adhesive dressing not to pull the catheter out. A catheter, which has migrated externally, should not be re-advanced to avoid introducing infection (RCN 2005). A repeat chest X-ray should be performed to establish the position of the distal tip of the catheter before any further drug administration.

Catheter damage

Catheter rupture or fracture is a rare but serious complication, which can occur in 'pinch-off syndrome' (Galloway and Bodenham 2004). 'Pinch-off syndrome' is a rare but potentially serious complication of subclavian access and occurs in up to 1% of all long-term devices (Andris *et al.* 1999, Polderman and Girbes 2002) (see Chapters 7 and 10). This must be treated acutely to prevent the intravascular portion from embolising, which occurs when there has been a complete fracture. Removal using radiological technique or surgical cut-down is required to prevent leakage of infused fluids into the subcutaneous tissues. The patient may feel general infraclavicular discomfort prior to shearing of the CVAD or there may be postural-related difficulty in injection whereby it is easier to inject when the patient is supine with the arm raised above the head. The first sign may be swelling due to extravasation of infusate. Any infusion must be stopped immediately and a chest X-ray/linogram ordered.

Catheter rupture may also occur when excessive force is used to flush a device or the wrong size of syringe. Syringe size is important as smaller syringes can create greater pressures (Conn 1993). Some manufacturers recommend that no syringe smaller than a 10 mL should be used. Catheter rupture may also be due to kinking which will be recognised when leakage occurs if the external portion is ruptured or by painful swelling on the chest wall if the internal portion is ruptured. The external portion of some types of catheters can be easily repaired, for example the Groshong™-valved catheters, but in the main it is usually advisable to replace the catheter. Repair of catheters may be contraindicated because of danger of introducing infection and/or air embolus.

Audit

A locally based audit should include patient identification data, presenting diagnosis and indication for catheterisation, date of catheter insertion, number of previous catheterisations, operator and department where catheter inserted, complications associated with the catheter, and date of and reason for removal. The CDC (2002) recommend that all centres should monitor their infection rates per 1000 catheter days to observe any changes or trends in infection rates, and be mindful of the emergence of any resistant bacterial patterns. Locally generated guidelines are useful to audit adherence to protocols and develop areas of care that require improvement.

Conclusion

CVADs insertion requires skilled operators, who operate regularly and according to strict aseptic protocol. However, if the CVAD is to last the duration of therapy, the aftercare and management must be of an equally high standard. Close liaison with the infection control team and microbiology departments is useful as is the development of specific teams to advise on the care of CVADs, as this has been shown to reduce the development of complications (Hamilton 2004).

References

Akl EA, Karmath G, Yosuico V *et al.* (2007). Anticoagulation for thrombosis prophylaxis in cancer patients with central venous catheters. *Cochrane Database of Systematic Reviews* (Online) 3:CD006468.

Andris D, Krzywda E, Shulte W *et al.* (1999). Pinch-off syndrome: a rare aetiology for central venous catheter occlusion. *Journal of Parenteral and Enteral Nutrition* 18:531–533.

Beathard GA (2003). Catheter management protocol for catheter-related bacteremia prophylaxis. *Seminars in Dialysis* 16:403–405.

Castagnola E, Molinari AC, Fratino G *et al.* (2003). Conditions associated with infections of indwelling central venous catheters in cancer patients: a summary. *British Journal of Haematology* 121:233–240.

Centres for Disease Control (CDC) (2002). Guidelines for the prevention of intravascular catheter related infections. Available at http://www.cdc.gov/ncidod/dhqp/gl_intravascular.html.

Cimochowski GE, Worley E, Rutherford WE *et al.* (1990). Superiority of the internal jugular over the subclavian access for temporary dialysis. *Nephron* 54:154–161.

Conn C. (1993). The importance of syringe size when using an implanted vascular access device. *Journal of Vascular Access Networks* 3:11–18.

Cook RJ, Ashton-Rendell W, Aughenbaugh GL *et al.* (2005). Septic pulmonary embolism: presenting features and clinical course of 14 patients. *Chest* 128:162–166.

Cornock M (1996). Making sense of CVCs. *Nursing Times* 92:30–31.

Couban S, Goodyear M, Burnell M *et al.* (2005). Randomized placebo-controlled study of low-dose warfarin for the prevention of central venous catheter-associated thrombosis in patients with cancer. *Journal of Clinical Oncology* 20:4063–4069.

Cox CE, Carson SS, Biddle AK (2003). Cost-effectiveness of ultrasound in preventing femoral venous catheter-associated pulmonary embolism. *American Journal of Respiratory and Critical Care Medicine* 168:1481–1487.

Craig D (2003). Clinical techniques. In *Conscious Sedation in Gastroenterology: A Handbook for Nurse Practitioners*, Skelly M, Palmer D (eds), Whurr Publishers, London, Chapter 4, pp. 50–67.

Crnich CJ, Maki DG (2002). The promise of novel technology for the prevention of intravascular device-related blood stream infections. II. Long term devices. *Clinical Infectious Diseases* 34:1362–1368.

Dougherty L, Lister SE (2004). Vascular access devices. In *Manual of Clinical Nursing Procedures*, Dougherty L, Lister S (eds), 6th edn. Blackwell Science, Oxford.

Fletcher SJ, Bodenham AR (1999). Catheter related sepsis: an overview. *British Journal of Intensive Care* 9:46–53.

Fletcher SJ, Bodenham AR (2000). Safe placement of central venous catheters: where should the tip of the catheter lie? *British Journal of Anaesthesia* 85:188–191.

Gabriel J, Bravery K, Dougherty L *et al.* (2005). Vascular access: indications and implications for patient care. *Nursing Standard* 19:45–54.

Galloway S, Bodenham AR (2004). Long-term central venous access. *British Journal of Anaesthesia* 92:722–734.

Goodwin M, Carlson S (1993). The peripherally inserted central catheter: a retrospective look at 3 years insertions. *Journal of Intravenous Nursing* 16:92–103.

Groeger JS, Lucas AB, Thaler HT *et al.* (1993). Infectious morbidity associated with use of long-term venous access devices in patients with cancer. *Annals of Internal Medicine* 119:1168–1174.

Hadaway LC (1998). Major thrombotic and nonthrombotic complications. Loss of patency. *Journal of Intravenous Nursing* 21:S143–S160.

Haller L, Rush K (1992). CVC infection: a review. *Journal of Clinical Nursing* 1:61–66.

Hamilton H (2004). Advantages of a nurse-led central venous access vascular service. *The Journal of Vascular Access* 5:109–112.

Heit JA, O-Fallon WM, Petterson TM *et al.* (2002). Relative impact of risk factors for deep vein thrombosis and pulmonary embolism: a population-based study. *Archives of Internal Medicine* 162:1245–1248.

INS (Intravenous Nursing Society) (2000). *Standards for Infusion Therapy*, INS and Becton Dickinson, Cambridge, MA.

Kelly C (1992). A change in flushing protocol of CVCs. *Oncology Nursing Forum* 19:599–605.

Krzywda EA (1999). Predisposing factors, prevention, and management of central venous catheter occlusions. *Journal of Intravenous Nursing* 22:S11–S17.

Laxson CJ, Titler MG (1994). Drawing coagulation studies from arterial lines: an integrative literature review. *American Journal of Critical Care* 3:16–22.

Lee AY (2005). Management of thrombosis in cancer: primary prevention and secondary prophylaxis. *British Journal of Haematology* 128:291–302.

Linares J, Sitges-Serra A, Garau J (1985). Pathogenesis of catheter sepsis: a prospective study with quantitative and semi-quantitative cultures of catheter hub and segments. *Journal of Clinical Microbiology* 21:357–360.

Lok-Charmaine E, Appleton D, Bhola C *et al.* (2007). Trisodium citrate 4% – an alternative to heparin capping of haemodialysis catheters. *Nephrology, Dialysis, Transplantation* 22:477–483.

MacDonald S, Watt AJ, McNally D *et al.* (2000). Comparison of technical success and outcome of tunnelled catheters inserted via the jugular and subclavian approaches. *Journal of Vascular and Interventional Radiology* 11:225–231.

Maki DG, Ringer M (1987). Evaluation of dressing regimes for prevention of infection with peripheral IV catheters. *JAMA* 258:2396–2403.

Mayo D, Pearson D (1995). Chemotherapy extravasation: a consequence of fibrin sheath formation around venous access devices. *Oncology Nursing Forum* 2:675–680.

McClelland DBL (2007). *Handbook of Transfusion Medicine*, 4th edn. UK blood transfusion and tissue transplantation services. Electronic version http://www.transfusionguidelines.org/index.asp?Publication = HTM&Section = 9&pageid = 1100.

MHRA (Medicines and Healthcare Products Regulatory Agency) (2005). *Medical Device Alert on All Brands of Needle Free Intravascular Connectors*, MDA/2005/030. London.

Mehall JR, Saltzman DA, Jackson RJ *et al.* (2002). Fibrin sheath enhances central venous catheter infection. *Critical Care Medicine* 30:908–912.

Mermel LA (2000). Prevention of intravascular catheter-related infections. *Annals of Internal Medicine* 132:391–402.

Morris P, Grace S, Glackin V *et al.* (1995). Audit of skin-tunnelled catheters in neutropenic patients. *Bone Marrow Transplantation* 15:S2, 168.

NICE (National Institute for Clinical Excellence) (2003). Infection control prevention of health-care associated infection in primary and community care. In *Clinical Guidelines 2*. DOH, London.

Olson K, Rennie RP, Hanson J *et al.* (2004). Evaluation of a no-dressing intervention for tunnelled central venous catheter exit sites. *Journal of Infusion Nursing* 27:37–44.

Passannante A, Macik BG (1998). Case report: the heparin flush syndrome: a cause of iatrogenic haemorrhage. *American Journal of Medical Science* 296:71–73.

Pearson ML (1996). Hospital infection control practices advisory committee. Guideline for prevention of intravascular-device-related infections. *Infection Control and Hospital Epidemiology* 17:438–473.

Pellowe C, Pratt RJ, Loveday H *et al.* (2004). The *epic* project. Updating the evidence base for national evidence-based guidelines for preventing healthcare associated infections in NHS hospitals in England: a report with recommendations. *British Journal of Infection Control* 5:10–16.

Polderman K, Girbes A (2002). Central venous catheter use. Part 1: mechanical complications. *Intensive Care Medicine* 28:1–17.

Pratt RJ, Pellow C, Harper P *et al.* (2001). The *epic* project: developing evidence-based guidelines for the prevention of healthcare associated infections. *Journal of Hospital Infection* 47:S1–S82.

Pratt RJ, Pellowe C, Wilson JA *et al.* (2007). Epic2: national evidence –based guidelines for preventing healthcare –associated infections in NHS hospitals in England. *Journal of Hospital Infection* 65:S1–S64.

Raad II, Hohn DC , Gilbreath BJ *et al.* (1994). Prevention of central venous catheter-related infections by using maximal sterile barrier precautions during insertion. *Infection Control and Hospital Epidemiology* 15:231–238.

Ray S, Stacey R , Imrie M *et al.* (1996). A review of 560 catheter insertions. *Anaesthesia* 51:981–985.

RCN (RCN IV Therapy Forum) (2005). *Standards for Infusion Therapy*. RCN, London.

Reynolds MG, Tebbs SE, Elliott TSJ (1997). Do dressings with increased permeability reduce the incidence of central venous catheter related sepsis. *Intensive and Critical Care Nursing* 13:26–29.

Rowley S (1997). Aseptic non-touch technique. *Nursing Times* 7:SV1–SVIII.

Schears GJ (2005). The benefits of a catheter securement device on reducing patient complications. *Managing Hospital Infection* 5:14–20.

Slichter-Sherrill J (2007). Platelet transfusion therapy. *Hematology/Oncology Clinics of North America* 21:697–729.

Tebbs ST, Trend V, Elliott TSJ (1995). The potential reduction of microbial contamination of central venous catheters. *Journal of Infection* 30:107–113.

Teichgräber UK, Gebauer B, Benter T *et al.* (2003). Central venous access catheters: radiological management of complications. *Cardiovascular and Interventional Radiology* 26:321–333.

Timsit JF, Farkas JC, Boyer JM (1998). Central vein catheter-related thrombosis in intensive care patients: incidence, risk factors and relationship with catheter-related sepsis. *Chest* 114:207–213.

Todd J (1998). Peripherally inserted central catheters. *Professional Nurse* 13:297–302.

Trerotola SO, Kuhn-Fulton J, Johnson MG *et al.* (2000). Tunnelled infusion catheters: increased incidence of symptomatic venous thrombosis after subclavian versus internal jugular venous access. *Radiology* 217:89–93.

Treston-Aurend J (1997). Impact of dressing materials on central venous catheter infection rates. *Journal of Intravenous Nursing* 20:201–206.

Vanherweghem JL, Dhaene M, Goldman M *et al.* (1986). Infections associated with subclavian dialysis catheters: the key role of nurse training. *Nephron* 4:116–119.

Vygon (2000). *Vygon Integrated Product Solutions; Mid to Long Term Vascular Access*. Vygon, Cirencester, UK.

Waghorn DJ (1994). Intravascular device associated systemic infections: a 2 year analysis of cases in a district general hospital. *Journal of Hospital Infection* 28:91–101.

Warkentin TE, Levine MN, Hayward CPM *et al.* (1995). Heparin induced thrombocytopenia in patients treated with low molecular weight heparin or unfractionated heparin. *New England Journal of Medicine* 332:1330–1335.

Wickham R, Purl S, Welker D *et al.* (1992). Long-term CVCs – issues for care. *Seminars in Oncology Nursing* 8:133–147.

Yamamoto AJ (2002). Sutureless securement device reduces the complications of peripherally inserted central venous catheters. *Journal of Vascular and Interventional Radiology* 13:77–81.

Chapter 15

Removal of central venous access devices

Sarah Drewett

Introduction

The removal of central venous catheters (CVCs) is commonplace within both hospitals and the community. There is much emphasis on the insertion and care of these devices, but very little focus, training or publications on their removal (Drewett 2000, Galloway and Bodenham 2003). There are potentially serious complications of such removal procedures (see Box 15.1).

It is worth noting that when a serious life-threatening complication occurs, associated with the removal of a CVC, the mortality rate is 57% due mainly to practitioner's lack of awareness of these rere but life-threatening complications (Kim et al. 1998). More minor complications, including patient anxiety and discomfort, are common.

This chapter aims to balance the inequality of knowledge and ensure that safe, high-quality patient care is given throughout the intravenous (IV) continuum from pre-insertion to post-removal.

This chapter focuses on removal of CVCs including assessments required preremoval, the most common complications of removal and their prevention, step-by-step procedures, with rationale, for the removal of the different types of CVCs.

Assessment of patients before removal

Due to the severity of complications that can occur during or after removal of a CVC, it is vital that a patient assessment is undertaken.

Reason for removal

The most basic, and often overlooked, question that needs answering prior to any removal is whether the CVC should be removed at all. Many practitioners are unfamiliar

---

Box 15.1 Complications associated with removal of CVCs:

Air embolism
Catheter fracture and embolism
Dislodgement or thrombus or fibrin sheath
Haemorrhage
Arterial complications – bleeding
Infection – local and systemic
Patient discomfort and anxiety
Inappropriately large or misplaced incisions
Poor cosmetic result

---

with a particular device and may ask for removal without attempting to treat a problem such as mild mechanical phlebitis in a PICC or an occlusion in a tunnelled, cuffed CVC. Although treatment has been discontinued, patient deterioration or further investigations subsequently may confirm a need to recommence treatment.

Some reasons for removal of a CVC are listed in the Box 15.2:

- *End of treatment.* Although CVCs should never be kept in place just in case they are required, there are always patients where the risk of keeping the CVC in situ are outweighed by the potential needs of requiring central venous access in the near future. For instance, after parenteral nutrition is completed to ensure the patient is tolerating an adequate diet, or after IV antibiotics to ensure blood cultures are negative and inflammatory markers remain low.
- *Proven and unresolved sepsis.* CVCs should generally only be removed if an infection is proven and unresolved (positive blood cultures from both the CVC and peripheral blood) and/or compromising the patient. Advice should be sought from a microbiologist regarding further management. In the presence of severe infection, empirical catheter removal for presumed infection may be appropriate. If a CVC is removed due to infection, the tip should be sent for microscopy, culture and sensitivity to ensure correct antimicrobial therapy is administered and rates of infection monitored.

Box 15.2 Reasons for removal of CVC:

End of treatment
Proven and unresolved sepsis
Device has exceeded recommended dwell time
Unable to repair, faulty/fractured device
Proven thrombosis
Unresolvable occlusion
Unresolvable phlebitis/thrombophlebitis

With PICCs mechanical phlebitis is a fairly common complication in the first week after insertion and can be easily mistaken for infection by an inexperienced practitioner.

- *Device has exceeded recommended dwell time.* Practitioners caring for and removing any IV device should be aware of its recommended dwell time. For example, a PICC is suitable for up to 1-year treatment, but is often thought to be suitable only for a month or two. If a CVC has been in for the recommended dwell time such as a non-tunnelled central line, and the patient continues to require central access, then future options need to be discussed and assessed prior to removal. Occasionally, if central access is problematic due to access or risk of complications, then a CVC may remain in situ for longer than the recommended dwell time or be rewired aseptically with a new CVC in the same position. For these options, the risk of infection needs to be balanced against the risks of attempting new central venous access.
- *Irreparable/faulty/fractured device.* The majority of long-term CVCs can be repaired if there is a fault/fracture in the external portion of the catheter. Faults internally need to be assessed carefully to minimise the risk of catheter embolisation during removal. All product faults should be reported to the manufacturer (with the batch number) and the MHRA (2005).
- *Proven thrombosis.* Before removing a device where there is a thrombosis in the blood vessel, medical advice should always be sought. A decision will need to be taken to:

  (a) Remove the device immediately and then anticoagulate the patient
  (b) Anticoagulate the patient and then remove (see 'blood tests' in Chapter 3)
  (c) Anticoagulate via the device and then remove the device (see 'blood tests' in Chapter 3)

- *Unresolvable occlusion.* Prior to removing an occluded CVC, drugs such as urokinase (blood occlusion) or alcohol (lipid occlusion) should be considered.
- *Unresolvable phlebitis/thrombophlebitis.* This complication only relates to PICCs and can be successfully prevented and treated (in the early stages) with the application of heat to the upper arm in order to dilate the vein housing the device. If a PICC does require removal due to this problem then this has been given as a reason for a PICC to become stuck during removal (Wall and Kierstead 1995) (see PICC removal procedure).

Blood tests

- *Biochemistry.* A potassium level outside of normal limits can cause the heart to be more susceptible to arrhythmias and should be rectified prior to removal of the CVC, if possible.
- *Haematology.* Platelet counts of greater than 50×10^9 L and a normal coagulation screen are required to reduce the risk of bleeding post-CVC removal. Anticoagulant therapy should be discontinued or titrated to ensure normal values. The activity of low-molecular-weight heparins is not easily monitored but effects may persist for

24 hours. For PICC removal, slightly altered coagulation or reduced platelet count is less restrictive as direct pressure over a prolonged period can be applied to the relatively smaller peripheral vein. The risk-benefits of stopping versus continuing full or partial anticoagulation should be balanced for each individual case.

Positioning and breathing during CVC removal

The supine position increases the central venous pressure (CVP) of an otherwise healthy person to higher than that of ambient pressure and the head down Trendelenburg position increases it further. Clinical dehydration leads to a low CVP increasing the risk of air embolism. A CVP higher than ambient pressure will prevent air aspiration into the venous system. If air is aspirated, greater quantities can be tolerated in the supine or Trendelenburg position as air can collect in the right ventricular apex and away from the pulmonary valve (Mennim *et al.* 1992).

Some patients are unable to lie completely flat or be placed in the head down Trendelenburg position, because it is either painful or for medical reasons. For instance, the Trendelenburg position may compromise those with raised intracranial pressure, recent eye surgery, severe heart disease or severe pulmonary disease. In such cases, the CVP can be raised for a few seconds by getting the patient to perform the Valsalva manoeuvre. The patient is asked to breathe in, and then forcibly expire with the mouth closed, the nose pinched and a closed glottis (larynx). This increases the intrathoracic pressure from a normal 3–4 to 60–70 mmHg, limiting the venous return of blood to the heart. As a result, the central veins become engorged. Falls in CVP can be reduced by asking a cooperative patient to exhale slowly or hold their breath.

Basic principles for removal of any CVC

The procedures for removal of each type CVC will follow, but there are some general principles including:

- Explanation of the procedure to the patient. This decreases patient anxiety and increases compliance with positioning and breathing techniques.
- Disconnection of infusion. This reduces the tug on the catheter aiding maintenance of sterility, controlled removal and preventing fluids within the device leaking into superficial tissues as the catheter is withdrawn.
- Strict aseptic technique – to reduce risk of infection at the exit site.
- Gentle traction if breakage of the device is to be avoided.
- New Point Gentle pressure to the vein exit site reduces the risk of air embolism until dressing applied.
- Gentle pressure to the exit site will reduce leakage of body fluids.
- Catheter inspection to ensure the entire device is intact.
- Dressing: the patient should not sit up until an occlusive dressing is applied to limit air entry (Drewett 2000).
- Observation of patient for 1 hour post-catheter removal should include: signs of discomfort, vital signs, colour and respiratory function (not PICC).

Complications of removal

It is worth noting that when a serious life-threatening complication occurs, associated with the removal of a CVC, the mortality rate is 57% due mainly to practitioners lack of awareness of these rare but life-threatening complications (Kim et al. 1998). These include:

Bleeding: If the catheter had been correctly sited in the venous system then bleeding should stop with appropriate pressure, but if the catheter is large-bore, skin sutures may be required to seal the incision (McCarthy *et al.* 1995). Bleeding into body cavities from veins may occur on removal if the vein has been damaged. In rare cases, the catheter may have entered or traversed an artery which may then lead to arterial bleeding on removal (Walden 1997) (see arterial puncture in Chapter 12).

Air embolus: See above and in Chapter 12.

Infection: Patients may develop a rigor within minutes of catheter removal if heavily infected. In this instance, infected clot is likely to be left behind as a continued focus for infection, so-called septic thrombophlebitis.

Catheter embolus (see Figure 15.1): Catheters may fracture if:

(a) excessive force is applied on removal
(b) sharp instruments are applied during dissection and surgical removal
(c) the catheter is already damaged as in pinch-off (see Chapter 7 and 10)

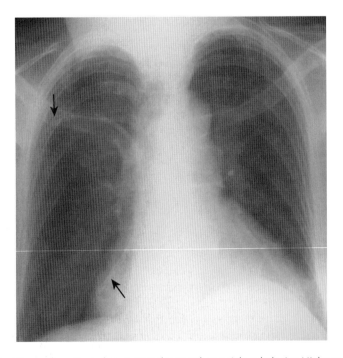

Figure 15.1 Chest X-ray of a patient after attempted removal on a right subclavian Hickman catheter by an inexperienced operator. The catheter has been cut during dissection of the cuff and has migrated inwards and its proximal end is lying within the subclavian vein and the distal end in the right atrium (arrows). The internal section was retrieved radiologically via the femoral vein.

Catheter will not withdraw from vein: Knotting or kinking may occur and occasionally catheters with side holes (e.g. apheresis catheters) get attached by organised thrombus to the vein wall, superior vena cava or right atrium and need surgery/radiology removal (see also Chapters 10 and 12).

A 'stuck' PICC may free with the following manoeuvres: straighten the arm, and thus the vein and apply heat to it. Apply slow, gentle traction whilst regrasping the catheter near the skin every few centimetres to allow for better control and a more even force along the length of catheter. This reduces the risk of the catheter breaking (Marx 1995). Avoid applying pressure to the vein and, therefore, the catheter touching the vein wall. If the PICC is still stuck tape the PICC under traction for 1/2 hour and reapply heat to reduce venous spasm.

Removal procedures

In addition to the above measures, tunnelled, cuffed CVCs and ports require surgical removal to free up the anchoring cuff or port membrane assembly.

Removal – tunnelled, cuffed catheters

See sequence of images a–l (Figure 15.2).

- If the catheter has been in less than 3–4 weeks, healing is delayed or the site is heavily infected then the cuff may not be fixed. In such cases, remove all sutures and attempt to pull out, under local anaesthetic, with judicious use of traction. If movable, the cuff will pull out with a series of gives as it passes through the tissues. If immovable, proceed to open removal to avoid breaking the catheter.
- Locate the subcutaneous Dacron cuff by observation or gentle palpation of the skin along the tunnel track. If unsure, gentle traction on the CVC produces skin puckering at cuff position. With most CVCs there is a measurement from a set external portion of line (e.g. hub or bifurcation) to cuff (see manufacturer's notes). Some practitioners advocate inserting a blunt-tipped probe up the track until resistance is felt, then lift the catheter/cuff towards the skin (Galloway and Bodenham 2003). If the cuff is at the exit site then there will be no movement of the catheter inwards when it is pushed along the line of the tunnel tract.
- Infiltrate all around the cuff with local anaesthetic.
- Make a small incision to one side of the cuff. The incision allows access to the cuff. The position of the incision avoids accidental severing of the catheter. If the cuff is at the exit site, then the cuff can be freed by slightly enlarging the exit site incision.
- Blunt dissection using mosquito artery forceps should be used to expose the cuff. Blunt dissection reduces bleeding and reduces risk of catheter damage and risk of embolisation. The cuff is the only portion of the CVC that adheres to the tissues although over time there will a fibrous membrane that grows around the whole length of CVC within the tissues. This sleeve membrane encloses the length of the catheter from the exit site to the vein, hence is a channel for bleeding or air intake.

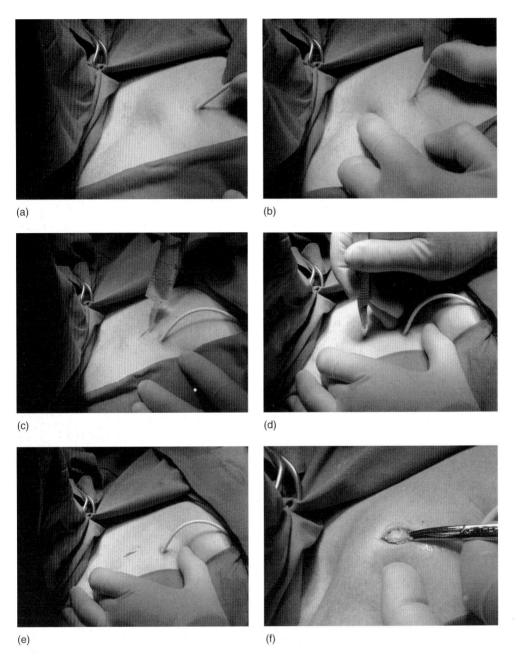

Figure 15.2 The images are arranged in blocks to show operating sequence (Hickman line removal images a–l). (a) The position of the anchoring cuff is found looking for skin puckering when the line is pulled. (b) The cuff can be felt by palpation when the line is pulled and pushed. (c) Local anaesthetic solution is infiltrated widely around the cuff site. (d) An incision has been made on the venous side of the cuff. (e) The incision is deepened with blunt dissection with artery forceps. (f) The cuff, catheter and attached tissue are pulled to the surface. Note the dull appearance of the white catheter which is obscured by fibrous tissue. (g) The adherent membrane is divided to reveal the bright white venous end of the line. (h) The catheter is pulled out of the vein. There should be minimal resistance to its removal. Press over the area of the tract leading to the vein to stop bleeding and prevent air entry. (i) The cuff is further dissected until it is free and can be pulled from the wound. (j) The catheter is then cut on the exit side of the cuff and both sections discarded. (k) The exit site is left to heal by granulation. (l) The cut down site is sutured with either an absorbable or a non-absorbable suture.

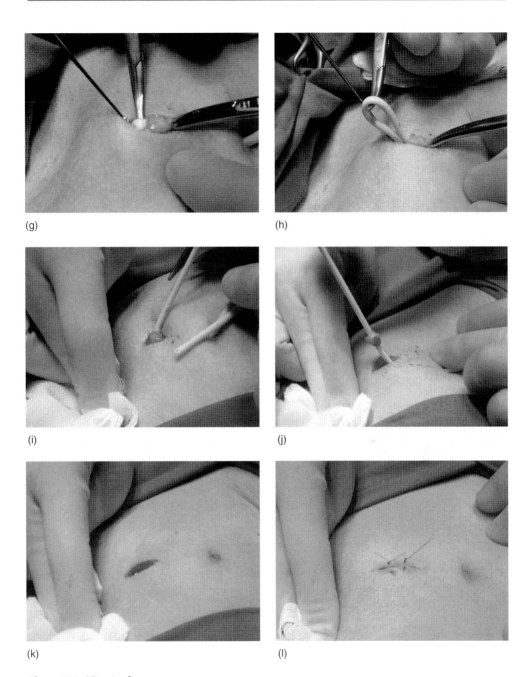

(g)

(h)

(i)

(j)

(k)

(l)

Figure 15.2 (*Contined*)

- This membrane is seen as a brown covering which dulls the bright white (or other colour) of the underlying catheter. It may require a firm rub with dry gauze or division with fine scissors to expose the catheter beneath. If trauma to the catheter does occur, it must be clamped atraumatically without delay to avoid air entry and/or haemorrhage (Drewett 2000).
- Free the catheter from the enclosing membrane on the venous side of the cuff. Ask the patient to hold their breath or perform a Valsalva manoeuvre, then withdraw the catheter in slow constant motion from the vein. There should be no resistance. As the catheter is removed, gentle pressure should be exerted on the vein exit site and the tunnel. This should be maintained for at least 5 minutes and until occlusive dressing has been applied.
- Whilst maintaining gentle pressure on vein exit site, remove the catheter from the vein and cut the catheter on the venous side of the cuff (send tip to microbiology if required). Then dissect out and remove the cuff. Remove lower/external portion of catheter from original skin exit site.
- Inspect catheter tip for completeness. An open-ended catheter should not have a ragged tip. A valve-tipped catheter (e.g. Groshong®) should have its radio-opaque tip intact. If in any doubt, an X-ray will confirm catheter fracture or embolism.
- The external portion of the catheter is not sterile and should not be pulled out through the surgical incision.
- Insert one or two skin sutures or surgical glue or paper sutures at the cuff dissection point.
- Leave exit site to granulate without suture.
- Apply sterile dressing to skin exit site and sutures. Cover both with an airtight dressing for at least 24 hours to prevent air entering while the track heals (Phifer *et al.* 1991).
- The patient should remain lying down, under observation for bleeding and other complications for at least 30 minutes.
- Document procedure and any further instructions.
- Skin sutures should be removed after 5–7 days (longer if patient has slower healing such as those on steroid therapy).

Subcutaneous ports are removed, usually in the operating theatre, by making an incision into the dense fibrous sac which forms around the port in the longer term. Once the sac is open, use a suitable instrument to grasp the port, e.g. a pointed towel clip through a suture hole in the base of the port. There are typically several anchoring sutures attaching the port to the tissues. There is usually dense scar tissue around the junction between port assembly and the catheter which also needs dissecting out prior to the catheter removal. The incision site is then sutured and pressure applied to the area to secure haemostasis.

Conclusion

Correctly performed removal procedures can be performed at the bedside safely and without significant discomfort to the patient. A sound knowledge of potential complications is required to avoid problems. The reader is reminded that, although this chapter gives the theoretical knowledge of how to remove each type of CVC, all new techniques require one-to-one training, practice and supervision to ensure high-quality care is maintained.

References

Drewett S (2000). Central venous catheter removal: procedures and rationale. *British Journal of Nursing* 9:2304–2315.

Galloway S, Bodenham A (2003). Safe removal of long-term cuffed Hickman-type catheters. *Hospital Medicine* 64:20–23.

Kim DK, Gottesman MH, Forero A *et al.* (1998). The CVC distress removal distress syndrome: an unappreciated complication of central venous catheter removal. *American Surgeon* 64:344–347.

Marx M (1995). The management of the difficult peripherally inserted central venous catheter line removal. *Journal of Intravenous Nursing* 18:246–249.

McCarthy PM, Wang N, Birchfield F *et al.* (1995). Air embolism in single-lung transplant patients after central venous catheter removal. *Chest* 107:1178–1179.

MHRA (Medicines and Healthcare Products Regulatory Agency) (2005). Medical alert on all brands of needle free intravascular connectors MDA/2005/030, issued 17 May 2005. Available at http://www.mhra.gov.uk/Safetyinformation/Reportingsafetyproblems/index.htm

Mennim P, Coyle CF, Taylor JD (1992). Venous air embolism associated with removal of central venous catheter. *British Medical Journal* 305:171–172.

Phifer TJ, Bridges M, Conrad SA (1991). The residual central venous catheter tract: an occult source of lethal air embolism: case report. *Journal of Trauma* 31:1558–1560.

Walden FM (1997). Subclavian aneurysm causing brachial plexus injury after removal of a sub-clavian catheter. *British Journal of Anaesthesia* 79:807–809.

Wall JL, Kierstead VL (1995). Peripherally inserted central catheters: resistance to removal: a rare complication. *Journal of Intravenous Nursing* 18:251–254.

Index